ALL THE LIVING AND THE DEAD

ALL THE LIVING AND THE DEAD

From Embalmers to Executioners, an Exploration of the People Who Have Made Death Their Life's Work

HAYLEY CAMPBELL

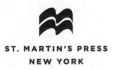

ST. MARTIN'S PRESS
NEW YORK

First published in the United States by St. Martin's Press, an imprint of
St. Martin's Publishing Group

www.stmartins.com

The Library of Congress Cataloging-in-Publication Data is available upon request.

ISBN 978-1-250-28184-5 (hardcover)
ISBN 978-1-250-28185-2 (ebook)

Our books may be purchased in bulk for promotional, educational, or business use.
Please contact your local bookseller or the Macmillan Corporate and Premium Sales Department
at 1-800-221-7945, extension 5442, or by email at MacmillanSpecialMarkets@macmillan.com.

Originally published in Great Britain by Raven Books, an imprint of Bloomsbury Publishing Plc

First U.S. Edition: 2022

10 9 8 7 6 5 4 3 2 1

Author's note

I have changed some details to protect the identities of the dead. The living, however, are as they came to me.

Life is tragic simply because the earth turns, and the sun inexorably rises and sets, and one day, for each of us, the sun will go down for the last, last time. Perhaps the whole root of our trouble, the human trouble, is that we will sacrifice all the beauty of our lives, will imprison ourselves in totems, taboos, crosses, blood sacrifices, steeples, mosques, races, armies, flags, nations, in order to deny the fact of death, which is the only fact we have.

— James Baldwin, *The Fire Next Time*

Contents

CONTENTS

ALL THE LIVING AND THE DEAD

Introduction

You aren't born knowing you will die. Someone has to break the news. I asked my dad if it was him, but he can't remember.

Some people remember being told: they have a moment they can pinpoint where life cleaved into before and after. They can remember the sound of a bird hitting the window, breaking its neck on the glass before the fall. They can recall the situation being explained to them as the limp, feathered body was peeled off the patio and buried in the garden, the dusty imprint of their wings lasting longer than the funeral. Maybe death came to you in the form of a goldfish or a grandparent. You might have processed mortality as much as you were able, or needed to, in the time it took for the fins to disappear in the swirl of a toilet bowl.

I don't have one of those moments. I can't remember a time before death existed. Death was just there, everywhere, always.

Maybe it began with the five dead women. Throughout my single digits, my dad – Eddie Campbell, a comic book artist – was working on a graphic novel called *From Hell*, written by Alan Moore. It's about Jack the Ripper and shows the full horror of his brutality in scratchy black and white. 'Jackarippy' was such a part of our lives that my tiny sister would wear the top hat to eat breakfast, and I would stand on tiptoes to study the crime scenes that were pinned to my dad's drawing board while trying to get him to agree to something Mum had said no to. There they were, the disembowelled women, the flesh torn from their faces and thighs. Next to them, the stark autopsy photographs, their sagging breasts and bellies, the pinched rugby-ball stitching from neck to groin. I remember looking up at them and feeling not shocked, but fascinated. I wanted to know what had happened. I wanted to see more. I wished the pictures were clearer, I wished they were in colour. Their situation was so removed from anything I knew of life that it was too *other* to be frightening – it was as alien to me there in tropical Brisbane, Australia, as the foggy London streets where they had lived. To look at those same photographs now is an entirely different thing – I see violence, the struggle and misogyny, the lost lives – but back then, I didn't have the emotional language to process something so terrible. It flew above my level of comprehension, but somewhere up there the bird hit the windowpane. Ever since then I have been peeling the body off the patio, holding it up to the light.

At seven I was much the same as I am now as a journalist: I put it down on paper in an attempt to figure it out. I sat beside my dad at an upturned cardboard box that I called my desk and I copied him, creating a felt-tip compendium of all the ways a human being could die, violently: twenty-four pages of people being murdered, pieced together from what I'd seen in movies, on TV, on the news, on his desk. They were cut up with machetes while they were sleeping, they were stabbed in the woods while hitchhiking, they were boiled by witches, buried alive, left to hang for the birds to eat. A drawing of a skull with the explanatory caption 'If someone chops your head off and your skin rots you look like this.' My dad bought a kidney from the butcher for a scene in the comic and laid it out on a handkerchief in the sitting room to paint. As it quickly turned rotten in the heat I drew the same scene beside him, only mine was more honest: it included the gathering cloud of flies. He kept all of my pages in a binder and proudly showed them off to horrified guests.

Death was outside the house too. We lived on a busy street where cats had shorter lifespans and turned up stiff in gutters; we lifted them by the tail like frying pans and buried them at dawn, quiet little ceremonies for cats we knew and cats we didn't. The walking route to school was altered in summer whenever a bird, usually a magpie, would die and decompose. It was something that wouldn't bear mentioning in cooler climates, but their decomposition was so fast in the soaring Australian heat that one bird could render a whole street impassable. Our headmaster would suggest avoiding that route until the smell of death had blown through it. I'd always walk the forbidden route to school, hoping to see the rancid bird so I could look it in the face.

Scenes of death had become familiar: I would often do my homework on the back of a photocopy of a drawing my dad had done, a spare piece of paper mindlessly picked off the top of the recycling pile. 'It's a dead prostitute,' I would tell my teacher, as she held up the offending pool of black blood and gore, speechlessly. 'It's only drawings.' Death seemed to be something that happened, and something that happened a lot. But I was being told it was bad, a secret, like I'd been caught trespassing. 'Inappropriate', as my teacher said on the phone to my parents.

It was a Catholic school. Our priest, Father Power – a mumbling Irishman who was, to me, impossibly old, yet could occasionally be seen leaping up and down on the contents of the skip in his priestly vestments in order to cram more rubbish inside it before the garbage collectors came – would sit us down once a week, at the front of the church, and speak to us plainly. He would pull out a chair and park it somewhere by the altar, using the stained-glass windows above to tell the story of Jesus hauling his cross to the place where he would die on it. One afternoon, Father Power pointed up at a red light to the left of the altar and said that when that light was glowing, God was in the house – it was powered by Him. I looked up at it, a red glowing bulb in an ornate brass cage, and asked why – if God was powering it – was there an extension lead running up the wall and down the chain that suspended it? There was a beat, a cleared throat, and the priest effectively said, 'No further questions at this time' before moving on to something else, forevermore considering me to be A Problem that required meetings with my parents (one proud, one embarrassed) and me being barred from ever getting involved in the bread and wine part of Mass.

It bothered me that he had tried to spin something magical and ghostly out of something electric, and from then on I regarded organised religion with suspicion. It seemed like a dodge, a panacea, some nice-sounding lies. Heaven felt a bit too easy, like a package holiday if you were good. I still had another dozen years of Catholic school to go, and the red bulb shone a warning light over everything religion offered in the way of an answer.

The first actual dead person I knew was my friend Harriet, who drowned rescuing her dog in a flooded creek when we were twelve. I remember almost nothing of the funeral, no eulogy, nor any of the teachers who came or if any of them cried. I don't remember where Belle the surviving black Labrador sat, or if she stayed at home. All I remember is sitting in a pew, staring at a closed white coffin, wanting to know what was in it. Every magician knows that sticking a closed box in the middle of a group of people is a recipe for sustained suspense – all I did was stare. My friend was there, mere feet away, but hidden from me. It was frustrating and hard to grasp the concept of someone being there, and then not, with nothing tangible to confirm it. I wanted to see her. I felt like I was missing something in addition to missing a friend. I felt like something was being kept from me. Wanting to see, and wanting to know the fact of it all but not being able to, was a block in front of my grief. Did she still look like my friend, or had she changed? Did she smell like the magpies?

I didn't fear death, I was captivated by it. I wanted to know what happened to the cats when we put them in the ground. I wanted to know why birds stink and what made them fall from the trees. I had books full of skeletons – human, animal, dinosaur – and would poke at my skin trying to picture my own. At home I had my questions answered, clumsily but honestly. I was praised for drawing it, and was shown, cat after heartbreaking cat, that it is an inevitability, sometimes messy, sometimes not. At school I was told to look away – from the birds, from the drawings, from my dead friend – and was given other images of death in every classroom and church: ones that told me death was temporary. To me, there was more truth in the photographs of the Ripper victims; no one told me they were coming back, but school said Jesus did, and would again. I was being handed a ready-made conceptual framework to replace the one I had begun to build for myself, that I had pieced together from experience. Through skirted questions and reactions to things I thought were simple facts, I was taught that death was taboo and something to fear.

We are surrounded by death. It is in our news, our novels, our video games – it is in our superhero comics, where it can be reversed on monthly whim. It is in the minutiae of the true-crime podcasts that saturate the internet. It is in our nursery rhymes, our museums, our movies about beautiful murdered women. But the footage is edited, the decapitated head of the journalist is pixelated, the words of the old songs are sanitised for modern youth. We hear about people burning to death in their flats, planes disappearing into the sea, men in trucks mowing down pedestrians, but it's difficult to comprehend. The real and the imaginary intermingle, become background noise. Death is everywhere, but it's veiled, or it's fiction. Just like in video games, the bodies disappear.

But the bodies have to go somewhere. Sitting there in that church, staring at my friend's white coffin, I knew that other people had pulled her from the water, dried her, carried her there; other people had cared for her where we could not.

On average, 6,324 people in the world die every hour – that's 151,776 every day, about 55.4 million a year. That's more than the population of Australia falling off the planet every six months. For most of those deaths in the Western world, there will be a phone call. Someone with a gurney will collect the body and transport it to the mortuary. If needed, another person will be called to clean the place where the body lay quietly decomposing until the neighbours complained, burning an outline into the mattress like a liquid victim of Pompeii. If there's no family, another person will be paid to clear the apartment of everything that once made up a lonely life: the shoes, the subscription magazines on the doormat, the piles of books that never got read after all, the food in the fridge that outlasted its owner, the things to be taken to auction, the things to be driven to the dump. At the funeral home, an embalmer might try to make the body look less dead, more sleeping.

They deal with the things we cannot bear to look at, or so we assume. Our sky falling is their routine.

Most of us have no relationship with the ordinary people who carry out this necessary work. They are kept at a distance, as hidden as death itself. We hear the news about the murders but never about the people who came to scrub the blood from the carpet and the arterial spray from the wall. We drive past the pile-ups but we don't hear about the people who trawl the gutters of the highway looking for body parts flung from the wreckage. When we mourn them on Twitter, we don't think about the people who unhooked our heroes from the doorknobs they hanged themselves from. They are the unfamous, unsung, unknown.

Death, and the people who make it their work, became a pre-occupation of mine that stretched across the years like a web. Daily, they encounter the truth that I was only able to imagine. The monster is always scarier when it's just footsteps in the air vents, but that's all we are offered with nothing real to ground it. I wanted to know what ordinary human death looked like – not photographs, not movies, not birds, nor cats.

If you are not a person like me, you will probably know someone who is. The one who makes you walk through old, ivy-covered cemeteries and tells you how this is the grave of a woman who stood too close to a fire and burned alive in her flammable dress; the one who tries to pull you into medical museums to stare at the white, bleached pieces of long-dead people whose eyes, if you've found the right jar, stare out. You may have wondered why they're drawn to such things. They – like Alvy Singer foisting a copy of Ernest Becker's The Denial of Death on Annie Hall – have wondered how on earth you couldn't be. I believe an interest in death is not just for the morbid: it has a mental gravitational pull unlike anything else. Becker considered death to be both the ender and the propeller of the world.

When people want answers they find them in churches, in therapy rooms, up mountains or on high seas. But I'm a journalist, and when your job is asking questions, you come to believe – or hope – that answers are in other people. My plan was to find those who work around death every day and ask them to show me what they do and how they do it — to explore not only the mechanics of an industry, but how our relationship to death plays out in their processes, how it forms a foundation for what it is that they do. The Western death industry is predicated on the idea that we cannot, or need not, be there. But if the reason we're outsourcing this burden is because it's too much for us, how do they deal with it? They are human too. There is no us and them. It's just us.

I wanted to know whether we are cheating ourselves out of some fundamental human knowledge by doing things this way. By living in this manufactured state of denial, in the borderlands between innocence and ignorance, are we nurturing a fear that reality doesn't warrant? Is there an antidote to the fear of death in knowing exactly what happens? In *seeing* exactly what happens? I wanted unromantic, unpoetic, unsanitised visions of death. I wanted the naked, banal reality of this thing that will come to us all. I didn't want euphemisms, or kind people telling me to talk about grief over tea and cake. I wanted to go to the root and grow my own thing from it. 'How can you be sure it is death you fear?' goes a line in Don DeLillo's *White Noise*. 'Death is so vague. No one knows what it is, what it feels like or looks like. Maybe you just have a personal problem that surfaces in the form of a great universal subject.' I wanted to shrink the size of death to something I could hold, something I could handle. I wanted to shrink it to the size of something human.

But the more people I spoke to, the more the questions were turned on me: What do you think you'll find — in this place where you needn't be? Why would you burn yourself up in this way?

There is a false security in believing that as a journalist you can stand there and report and be the interloper in all situations, unaffected, the detached observer. I thought I was invulnerable; I was not. I was right in that I was missing something, but I was naive as to how far down the damage goes, how much our attitude towards death affects our everyday lives — how much it stunts our ability not only to understand, but to grieve, when things fall apart. I've finally seen what real death is like, and the transformative power of seeing is almost beyond words. But I found something else there too, in the dark. Just like with dive watches and childhood bedroom ceilings stickered with stars, you have to turn the light off to see the glow.

The Edge of Mortality

'The first dead body you see should not be someone you love,' she said.

About fifty of us are in a large room at University College London, holding a 'wake' for a long-dead philosopher on his 270th birthday. His severed head, on show for the first time in decades, is in a bell jar by the Budweisers. Down the hall, his skeleton sits in a glass box as usual, dressed in his own clothes, his gloved skeletal hand perched on his walking stick, with a wax head where his real one was supposed to go, back before the plan for preservation went wrong. Students nearby pay him as much attention as they would a piece of furniture.

Between annual checks to note new stages of decrepitude, Jeremy Bentham's real head is usually locked away in a cupboard, and nobody gets to see it. Dr Southwood Smith, executor of Bentham's will and dissector of his body, had tried to preserve it so it looked untouched, extracting the fluids by placing the head under an air pump, over sulphuric acid. But the head turned purple and stayed that way. He admitted defeat and contacted a wax artist to create a fake one, while the real head was hidden. But three years prior to tonight's wake, a shy academic in charge of Bentham's care had shown it to me for a piece I was writing. We peered at his soft blond eyebrows and blue glass eyes as his dried skin filled the room with the smell of beef jerky. He told me that when Bentham was alive he used to keep his future glass eyeballs in his pocket, getting them out at parties for a laugh. Here they were now, 186 years after his death, wedged in leathery eye sockets, looking out on a room full of people gathered to talk about society's backward attitude towards death.

Bentham was an eccentric philosopher – some of his ideas would land him in prison today, or at least get him thrown off the university campus – but he was ahead of the curve on many things. As well as being a champion of animal rights and women's rights, he believed in gay rights at a time when homosexuality was illegal, and he was one of the first to donate his body to science. He wanted to be publicly dissected by his friends, and everyone here is the kind of person who would have gone to watch. Already we had heard from Dr John Troyer, the director of the Centre for Death and Society at the University of Bath, who talked about growing up in a funeral home, in a family where death was not taboo, another house where death was everywhere. Then a gentle palliative care doctor encouraged us to talk about our own death before it happens, to have our wishes (however mad) in place before we go, like Bentham had done. Finally, Poppy Mardall, a funeral director in her mid-thirties, stood up and told us that the first dead body you see should not be someone you love. She said that she wished she could bring schoolchildren to her mortuary to confront death before they have to. *You need to be able to separate the shock of seeing death from the shock of grief*, she said. She thanked us for listening and sat down, the beer bottles clinking on the table.

In all of my thinking about death, I had never considered this idea – that you could deliberately separate these specific shocks to save your own heart. I wondered what I would be like now, if I had met her as a child and she had shown me what I had wanted to see. I was always curious about what dead bodies looked like, but I assumed that when I saw someone dead it would be because I had known them in life. It's not like anonymous dead bodies were easy to come by – I hadn't even been shown the one I did know, nor did I see the ones that came in the years after: more school friends (cancer, suicide), four grandparents (natural causes). The psychological impact of losing someone you love and confronting the physical reality of death at the same time, and the tangled mindfuck that might be, was not something I thought I could swerve.

A couple of weeks after Bentham's wake, I was sitting on a wicker chair in a brightly lit room in Poppy's funeral home, an old brick gatehouse by the entrance to Lambeth Cemetery. Colourful Easter eggs filled a small bowl in the centre of the table, poppy flower decals stuck to the vast Victorian windows. Outside, snow was gathering on the sandalled feet of a stone Jesus. Lambeth Cemetery is less grand than the famous seven that form a ring around London – Kensal Green, West Norwood, Highgate, Abney Park, Brompton, Nunhead and Tower Hamlets – those large garden cemeteries built in the nineteenth century to deal with the overcrowded parish churchyards in the middle of the growing city. Unlike them, Lambeth has no extravagant mausoleums, no grand promenades, no tombs as big as houses to flaunt the wealth of its dead inhabitants. It is practical, small, unpretentious, and so is Poppy. She's easy to talk to – you can imagine her being a therapist, or a good mother. I had been so struck by what she said in her speech that I wanted to hear more. She clearly thought of her role as much more than a job. Also, as I had never seen a dead body before, in person – decapitated philosophers not withstanding – I wondered if she might be the one to show me. It's not a favour you can ask of most people.

'We don't open the fridge doors just to see people,' she says, matter-of-factly. 'I want us to be careful with the behind-the-scenes thing – it's not like a museum. But if you had a spare couple of hours, you could come back and help get someone ready for their funeral. Then you're actually having an engagement with the body, rather than just seeing a load of dead people.' I blinked at her. I didn't think she'd actually say yes, let alone invite me to be involved in someone's funeral preparation. I'm here because she said it's something she wishes she could share, of course, but even so, there are some doors that have been closed for so long it can seem impossible to imagine them opening. 'You would be very welcome,' she insisted, filling my stunned silence.

In the UK, a funeral director needs no licence to handle the dead, as they do in America. Here, all of Poppy's staff come from places other than the funeral industry: Poppy herself used to work at the auction house Sotheby's, until she felt the meaninglessness of her work life bearing down on her. Aaron, who now runs the mortuary, a short walk across the cemetery from where we sit, used to work at the greyhound track nearby; the body collection van driver, Stuart, is a firefighter, and says that working here part-time is like going back for the ones he couldn't save. Poppy said I could come and be trained like they were, as if I was starting work here too.

'Had you seen a dead body before you became a funeral director?' I asked.

'No,' she says. 'Isn't that insane?'

I try to figure out the path between hectic art auction house and running a funeral home and I cannot begin to make a guess. 'I meet people who have a much clearer reason for doing this kind of thing,' she says, laughing. 'For me, it wasn't like that at all.' The way she tells it, the route may have been winding, but her motivation is lucid, even if she couldn't see it at the time.

It was Poppy's love of art that got her into the world of auction houses – first Christie's, then Sotheby's – and it was the fun that kept her there: the adrenaline, the socialising, the unpredictable nature of where in the world she could end up. 'A guy called saying he thought he had a Barbara Hepworth sculpture in rural Texas, so the next day I was on a flight,' she says, picking an example she says wasn't even particularly unusual. 'I was twenty-five, I had buckets of responsibility, it was fun, fun, fun. But quite quickly, I felt like there was a vacuum of meaning.' Her parents, one a social worker and the other a teacher, had instilled in her an obligation to help people in need, and her job at Sotheby's was – while exciting – not fulfilling that need in herself. 'From a sustenance point of view, I couldn't live off selling paintings,' she says.

In her spare time she became a Samaritan, volunteering to answer the phones at the charity that provides emotional support to those feeling lost or suicidal. But as her job became busier, as the travel kept her further away from home, her shifts would get missed or moved. 'It made me very sad. I spent about two years just not having the answer. I was having a sort of quarter-life crisis.' She knew she wanted to engage with regular people on the frontline of existence, to do something that *mattered* – birth, love or death, it wasn't important which – but she couldn't figure out how, or what, until life began to make the decision for her.

The fact that everyone we love will one day die often doesn't dawn on us until something bad happens. Poppy hadn't processed it herself until both of her parents got cancer diagnoses in quick succession. 'Our family is super open about everything,' she says. 'My mum was rolling condoms onto bananas when I was five, which didn't make any sense to me, she just loved the idea of breaking taboos. But we didn't really talk about death. We'd never had that discussion, or not in a way that I understood it. I was twenty-seven when my dad got sick, and it was genuinely the first time I realised he was ever going to die.'

This realisation arrived in the maelstrom of her crisis about her job. Conversations long ignored were now being had. When it was clear that both of her parents were going to survive, she saved some money, quit the art world and went to Ghana for a break. There she got typhoid and nearly died too.

'Jesus Christ,' I say.

'I know! Anyway, I was sick for eight months, so it gave me this very long period of inactivity and a chance to think. The job I would have picked if I hadn't got typhoid would have been a lot safer. This,' she says, motioning to the funeral home around us, 'was definitely the craziest thing on my list.'

Funeral directing was on the list not only because it involves one of the big life events Poppy wanted to be part of, but because her mother had made it clear what she did and did not want in a funeral. Researching options as her parents became sick, Poppy had seen how stuck in the past the industry was, how little room there was for personalisation. The shiny black hearses and top hats, the stilted formal processions, were not right for a family like hers. Now she wanted to play a part in changing the world of death, but even she didn't know what, exactly, she meant by that. It wasn't until she started her training by shadowing existing funeral directors, at the tail end of her own sickness, when the fatigue had lifted enough to leave the house, that she understood what she had been missing. She stood in a mortuary and saw death for the first time in all its unterrifying banality, and it struck her that she was angry. She had been forced to face the idea of death – in her family, in herself – without ever knowing what it looked like.

'It would have been really helpful to have had dead people in my life before then,' she says. With two small children, Poppy likens the intensity of her fear to pregnancy. 'If I was nine months pregnant and I was going to give birth any minute, but I'd never seen a child under the age of one, it would definitely be more scary for me. I would be giving birth to something that I'd never seen before, and could not imagine.'

I ask about the bodies we do imagine: the ones that aren't just pale and sleeping, the decayed, bloated corpses our minds serve up for us. They do exist. Should there ever be a limit placed on what the family can see? 'Suggesting people shouldn't see the body comes from a good place of care and concern, but I think it gets very patriarchal and patronising about what people can cope with,' she says. 'Not everyone needs to see the body, but for some it is a primal need.'

There was a man, years ago, who came to Poppy with a question. His brother had drowned and had been in water for a long time – long enough that every funeral home he spoke to said that the body could not be viewed. 'The first thing he asked us was, *Would you stop me from seeing my brother?* It was a test. He was asking, *Are you on my side or are you not on my side?* It's not our role to tell people what they can and cannot do. We're not here to force a transformational experience on people who don't want it. Our role is to prepare them, to gently give them the information they need in order to make an empowered decision. You don't know them; you don't know what the right decision is.' The man got to see his brother one last time.

She tells me when I come back the mortuary will be beautiful, because it has to be: it's critical that she keeps the dead somewhere lovely because she wants to let the living in. 'Lots of people who

visit our mortuary say things like, "Why have you put the mortuary here? This is the most inspiring space." I just feel like that is
the point.'

Back I went. The snow had long since melted.

§

This is not how I expected a mortuary to smell. I had pictured
a room without windows, squeaking linoleum floors, the stench
of bleach and rot. I had predicted an assault of fluorescent strip
lights that buzz and blink, not a place bathed in warm spring sunlight making everything shine and glitter, steel and wood alike.
I'm standing by the door in a disposable plastic apron, my hands
sweating inside nitrile gloves. Roseanna and Aaron, wearing
matching green fleeces and the same crinkling plastic as me, are
readying the room: she's rolling a gurney out from the corner,
he's making neat notes in a black ruled logbook. A shopping bag
of folded clothes sits by the sink, waiting to be worn for the last
time. I lean awkwardly against a shelving unit of polished wooden
coffins, trying not to get in the way. It smells of pine.

There are thirteen bodies in the house today, their names written
by different hands on small whiteboards stuck to the heavy doors
of the mortuary fridge. Soft-lit lamps dangle from the crossbeams
above, but it's so bright outside they were likely only switched on
by habit. Everything that is not metal is made of wood. The door
of the cupboard by the sink is ajar; inside, a bottle of Chanel No. 5
stands by bamboo headrests. The new coffins stand upright in
their rows, catching the light, their corners bound in cling film
for protection from bumps. There are two wicker caskets acting as
bookends, and on a high shelf, a Moses basket for babies – blue-
checked print, small, waiting. A picnic basket, but not.

It wasn't always a mortuary. Below the arched, lead-lined
window, the wall of white refrigerators hum low and steady where
the altar might have been back when this was a burial chapel,
before it fell into thirty years of disrepair, abandoned but still
standing in the middle of this cemetery in south London. It was
rescued from slow dilapidation by Poppy when she was a new

independent funeral director in need of a place to house her dead. Long ago, the dead would spend the night before their funeral in this building. Poppy has restored it to its original use.

She's not here today with me – I've been left in the hands of two trusted employees. Poppy has had her experience of meeting the dead, and now she's leaving me to mine. But as I look around the room, her presence is everywhere: it is practical, unpretentious, welcoming. I see a kitchen sink and bench in one corner, all that is required for the kind of body preparation done here, and remember her telling me, as the snow fell outside, that there is no embalming done on the premises. 'We want to provide what's useful for the public, and when we set up I wasn't sure that embalming is happening for the family's sake,' she said. 'I think it's happening because of how funeral directors are structured.' She explained that not every high-street funeral home has their own wall of fridges, not everyone has space like she does, so bodies are kept in a central depot and ferried to and from other locations as required. If a family wishes to view the body, the chances of it needing to be transported and therefore out of refrigeration for a period of hours – maybe ten, maybe twenty-four – are high. Embalming, which preserves the body and allows it to be kept at room temperature for a longer period without decomposing, makes the admin of moving bodies easier on the funeral home – it gives them more time. Here, if a family specifically asks for a body to be embalmed, Poppy would facilitate it, and the process would take place elsewhere. But in the six years she's been running her business, she is yet to be convinced that it is as important as some claim it to be. She is, as always, ready for someone to change her mind.

In these fridges, everything that needs to be done has been done. All the medical interventions have been completed, the autopsy incisions sewn up, all the evidence has been gathered and weighed. Here they become people again, not a patient or a victim or a fighter in a battle against their own body. Here they are finished, just waiting to be washed and dressed, then buried or burned.

I remember the filmmaker David Lynch, in an interview, talking about visiting a mortuary when he was a young art student in Philadelphia – he had met the nightwatchman in a diner and asked if he could come see it. Sitting on the mortuary floor, the door closed behind him, it was the stories in all of these bodies that got to him: who they were, what they did, how they got there. Like him, it's the scale of it, both large and small, that sweeps over me like a wave: all of these people, all of these individual libraries of collected experience, all of them ending here.

The fridge door opens with a clunk and a body is pulled out on a tray that slots into the gurney, raised by a hydraulic pump with a loud metallic hiss to waist height. The fridge hums louder, the machine whirring to correct the temperature rise. Aaron wheels the body into the centre of the room and looks at me, backed up against the coffins, fidgeting with my apron. From where I stand, all I can see is the dome of a shaved head resting on a white pillow. His name is Adam.

'We need to remove his T-shirt, the family want to keep it,' Aaron says. 'Could you come hold his hands?'

I step forward and take the man's cold hands in mine, raising his long, thin arms above his body so his T-shirt can be inched over his bony shoulders. Holding them there, I lock on to his face, on his half-open sunken eyes that clung to the corners like oysters in their shells. Aaron will tell me later that they always try and shut the eyes when people arrive here – the longer you leave it, the drier the eyelid becomes, the harder it is to move and manipulate. These eyes are not round like marbles, they are deflated, like whatever life was there had leaked out. You can look into the eyes of the dead and find nothing, not even a familiar shape.

Adam had been clutching a daffodil and a framed family photograph in the refrigerator – that was how he was positioned when he had been collected from his home, where he had died in his bed – but both were lifted off his chest and placed to the side, out of the way, while I wasn't looking. I think, later, that this was the only chance I would get to see this man alive, but I was so fixated on Adam, as he was then, that I missed it. I wish I had seen it, but

I can't blame myself: this was the first dead person I had ever seen, and here I was holding his hands.

I had wanted to see what death looked like, and Adam looked dead. Unembalmed, naturally dead. He had been in these refrigerators for two and a half weeks and it showed, even though in terms of decomposition, his had been a best-case scenario – the interval between his death and cold storage had been kept to a minimum. His mouth was half open, just like his eyes. I could not tell what colour they had been in real life, or if any of the colours he was now would relate to anything that he looked like a month ago. He was a sickly yellow from jaundice, but it wasn't the brightest colour on his body. As his T-shirt slid over his head, I could see that each protruding rib was highlighted in an even brighter yellow, contrasting with the lime green of his stomach and the darker black-green in the spaces between each jutting bone. The stomach is usually the first place to show signs of decomposition, filled as it is by design with bacteria, but I didn't know that death, something so emotionally black, could be so bright: the sight of microbial life taking over a human one is almost luminous. His back was purple from where the blood had pooled; no longer pumped around the body by the heart, it is left to coagulate and darken where it stands. His skin was bunched in places from being stored in a position a live person would have wriggled out of for comfort, but without life and movement to keep skin supple, a fold remains a fold, an indent an indent. His legs were yellow-white at the top and purplish behind the knee. He wasn't old. Forties, maybe. His family wanted his shirt back. It was blue.

I couldn't tell if his ribs had stuck out like that in life, or if he had – like his gaunt face – generally sunk. The muscles on his slim legs said he was a fit man, possibly a runner. You don't need to know how someone died when you're only there to dress them, and you rarely find out, but the fentanyl painkiller patches on his arm and sticky outlines on the skin where previous patches had been removed suggested a long illness. Roseanna gently rubs at the places where the patches used to be, trying to get rid of the glue. 'We remove as much as we can without damaging them,' she says.

'If we start removing a plaster and someone's skin starts to come off, we'll just leave it.' She tells me that as much as possible, they make all evidence of hospitals and medical intervention vanish. Nobody needs to go to their grave wearing compression socks and the disconnected end of an IV drip.

The shopping bag is fetched from the sink and emptied onto the bench. Trainers, bunched-up socks, grey boxer shorts with a hole in the crotch. All of his clothes were old and casual, picked out of his closet by his family. Everything was worn except for his trainers, which looked like they'd been owned for maybe a week at most. I flip them over in my gloved hands and wonder when he had bought them, whether he felt well enough to believe he had time to warrant new shoes. What's the joke about the old guy not buying green bananas?

Aaron removes Adam's underwear, carefully keeping a sheet over the groin, trying to keep the body covered at all times out of respect. 'After we remove the underwear, we check he's clean. If he's not, we clean him.' We roll him on his side, Aaron checks the situation, we roll him back. Roseanna takes one side of his fresh underwear and I take the other, each of us edging them up his yellow legs inch by inch. His skin is so cold I comment on it, then feel stupid. 'After a while you become accustomed to them being cold,' says Aaron, reassuringly. 'Then you go on a home collection for somebody who's just died and they're still warm. It's ... quite a strange feeling.' He shoots a look like the warmth is unnerving, an unwelcome sign of life in a situation where a drop in temperature helps him mentally separate the living from the dead. Here, the fridges are cooled to 4 degrees Celsius.

We roll Adam on his side again, edge the boxer shorts up. We roll him the other way and do the same. Dressing the dead is all pretty self-explanatory, you're just dressing a man who isn't helping. 'I like the way they haven't bought new or fancy clothes for his funeral,' I say. 'They're probably his favourites,' says Roseanna. It's hard not to piece together a personality from the scant details provided in a shopping bag.

Aaron asks me to lift Adam's head in my hands so he can slip the clean T-shirt on. I'm leaning over the gurney, holding the sides of his face as if I'm about to kiss him, thinking, *Unless somebody hauls him out of his coffin tomorrow, I'm the last woman on earth to hold him this way. How did we get here?*

'Place your hand up through the trouser leg and take hold of his foot,' directs Aaron next. With his light blue jeans bunched over my wrist, I grip his toes. As we move him, rolling one way and then the other to pull the jeans up, trapped air escapes from Adam's lungs with a sigh. There's a smell of slightly-off chicken, raw, still cold.

It's the first smell of death I've encountered today and it's instantly recognisable. Denis Johnson wrote about this smell, in a story called *Triumph Over the Grave*: he said that ethyl mercaptan, the first in a series of compounds brought out in the process of putrefaction, is routinely added to gas to make leaks detectable by scent. The practice originated in the 1930s, after workers noticed vultures in California would circle the thermal drafts around leaks in pipelines. They ran tests on their product to see what had attracted these birds, ordinarily lured by the odour of decay, and found trace amounts of this compound. The gas companies decided to amplify the effect, deliberately adding larger quantities of something that happened accidentally, so that humans could smell it too. It's a perfect Denis Johnson fact, a writer whose stories could seem nihilistic and bleak but could end on a line of strange hope. He found the life in the smell of death, the hope in birds ordinarily cast as omens of doom; he found that something so funda-mental in our fear — death and decay — could be quietly repurposed to save our lives. I thread Adam's belt through the loops, buckling it at a belt hole only recently broken in.

We line up the coffin on another gurney beside him and pos-ition ourselves to move him. Each of us grips the waterproof calico sheet under his body — a legal requirement in unsealed wicker coffins — and we lift him in. His head is cocked quizzically on his pillow, the coffin just long enough. He'll only stay like that for a night. Tomorrow, he'll be cremated. This whole person will no longer exist.

Aaron places the photo and the daffodil back on Adam's chest — the yellow flower has lost its spring perkiness and slumps against the fabric of his clean T-shirt, this one crisp white. We lay his long fingers over the stem. Dressed and packed in his coffin, we slide him back into the fridge, on a shelf adjusted to accommodate the height of it. Beside him, in the dark, more heads rest on pillows beside rosary beads, flowers, picture frames. A single crocheted Rasta cap. We only get one ending, one ritual – whatever it might be – and I was part of Adam's. Aaron writes his name on the door and I stand silent with a lump in my throat. I've never felt more privileged and honoured to be anywhere in the world.

§

The artist and AIDS activist David Wojnarowicz wrote in his memoir Close to the Knives how the experience of his friends dying of AIDS in accelerating numbers, with no government action to stop it, left him feeling acutely aware of himself being alive. He saw, as he put it, the edge of mortality. 'The edge of death and dying is around everything like a warm halo of light sometimes dim some-times irradiated. I see myself seeing death.' He felt like a runner who suddenly finds himself in solitude among trees and light, and the sight and sounds of friends are way back in the distance.

On the Tube home from the mortuary, I am aware of my own breathing, conscious of the fact that there are people lying in fridges who cannot. I am aware of the mechanism of life: the fact that this meat machine moves, somehow, and then it doesn't. I look at people in the Tube carriage and I see death. I wonder if they own the clothes they will die in, I wonder who will take care of them when they are dead. I wonder how many people hear the clock tick as loudly as I do right now.

I go to the gym, but this time it feels different. Usually I come here to quieten my mind; today it is irretrievably deafening. The sound of the living is unbelievably loud when you've been in the company of the dead. In a spin class I hear people gasping, heaving and shouting. It's the sound of survival, the impermanent and unlikely state of being alive. Everything is more vivid than usual, every sense heightened. These vocal cords being used, these hearts beating and lungs inflating, monotonous and vital. I feel the physical warmth radiating off strangers, fogging up the windows. I feel the blood rushing through my veins. 'Nobody dies in spin class!' shouts the instructor. 'Push yourself to failure!' I'm thinking that one day all of these bodies will fail and everything will fall silent but for the hum of the mortuary fridge.

I lie on my back in the heat of the sauna, each bench barely bigger than the tray that held Adam, and I make one of my arms go limp. I pick it up by the hand and imagine someone is peeling the T-shirt off my dead body. But it doesn't matter how hard I try, I can never fully relax my arm to the point where it's a dead weight. It doesn't feel the same. Lying next to me, a sweating, live woman tells me that she's started Botoxing her feet. Botox your feet and you can numb the pain enough to stand in heels all day, she says. When did we forget that pain is a warning, a scream from the voiceless parts of our bodies saying it needs help, something is wrong, something requires our attention? *I've got this great way of dealing with things that might be damaging me – I just switch off the notifications.* I drop my arm again. Today was the first death I've experienced where none of it was mitigated or obscured in some way, none of the notifications were turned off. It was all there. It felt real and meaningful, like I would be missing something crucial if I put any of it on mute. I think of Adam holding his faded daffodil, and how the bulbs, if eaten, can numb the nervous system and paralyse the heart.

The Gift

In a chilled room off the lab, a small body lies on a metal table, a towel draped over her recently shorn head. 'I only know one haircut,' says Terry Regnier, whose own hair is neat and grey, combed back like Elvis, with matching sideburns and a moustache I would file under both 'trucker' and 'porno'. 'Nobody's studying the hair. Plus, one of my bigger fears is that somebody would know the donor. Shaving the head helps them become less recognisable.' Somewhere, echoing off cold steel, I can hear a radio playing. Terry reaches behind some equipment and flips the switch, killing ELO's 'Sweet Talkin' Woman'.

For weeks after dressing the dead man at the funeral home, I kept thinking about what a waste death is. A body that has spent years growing, repairing itself, retaining knowledge of viruses and diseases and immunity, is just buried or burned. It should always be your choice to do whatever you like with your body, but seeing them all there in the glimpses through the refrigerator door, their heads resting on pillows, waiting to disappear, felt to me like there could be something more to this. I don't believe our sense of meaning or value in life or death should come solely from a place of utility, but there is space for it and always – even in a time of 3D prints and virtual simulations – a need for it. I wanted to see what happened to the bodies that people donated to science, the ones that didn't go straight to the grave or the crematorium, the ones that had a second life in places like this, at the Mayo Clinic in Minnesota. And I wanted to know whether a sea of anonymous dead faces would change the nature of the job for whoever was caring for them. Did knowing a dead person's name make any difference in how you treat them or what it means to care for them? There is no shopping bag of clues beside a medical cadaver. There isn't one now, beside the new arrival.

She is hooked up to the embalming machine, a black rubber pipe disappearing under another towel towards her upper thigh, pumping a combination of alcohol, glycerine (a moisturiser), phenol (a disinfectant) and formalin (a preservative) through her vascular system. It will add 30 per cent to her weight in fluid; unlike in a funeral situation, where a body rarely needs to be around longer than a few weeks, this body will need to be usable for about a year, so here they go overboard. She'll look bloated, shrinking over the months as she dehydrates. Beneath her head, a ceramic bowl fills with the blood pushed out of her veins by the incoming embalming fluid. It's dark red, almost black, some congealed into clots. I can't smell the blood, or the woman: the room smells like steel and formalin, that same chemical odour from the high-school biology lab, the one that engulfed you if you ever took the lid off a jarred toad. Her face and body are covered, but pale winter skin is visible on her liver-spotted arms. She had only died that morning, so she hadn't yellowed or greyed or greened. In her life she'd only had a gallbladder removed. Her whole body was good to use.

I walk around to the other side of the table, brushing up against a bone saw. One hand peeps out from beneath the fabric that covers her, nails painted bright orange, the nail on the ring finger a glittering gold. Terry used to remove the nail polish, but after hearing one student speak about her cadaver's nails, he stopped. For the student, the painted nails were the thing that humanised this inanimate meat. It said to her: this is a person who lived and died and gave you this gift to learn from. Terry never touched another bottle of nail polish remover. 'I've had guys come in and their grandkids have done their fingernails. I'm leaving that on too.'

After a body is embalmed and before it is assigned to an educational course, Terry allows it to lie in state for two to three months to allow the chemicals to firm the tissues. The refrigeration and delay helps kill any harmful bacteria, on top of the safety precaution of rejecting donors if there is infectious concern, like HIV, hepatitis or bird flu. This lady with the gold and orange nails won't be meeting her students for a while yet. When she does, parts of her will be thawed according to need. If she is required on a course that studies the airways in the neck, they will pack the rest of her in dry ice, thawing the head and neck alone. Extremities and heads take a day to thaw; torsos, depending on the size, more like three. 'We try to keep it as pristine as possible, yet thawed enough for their use. It's cold enough in Minnesota,' he chuckles. 'We don't want the tissue to be frozen as well.'

Terry opens the huge silver door on the right, revealing a cool room with multiple shelving units, four shelves high. There's a black plastic chest on the top shelf, empty for now but used as a transport system for torsos. There's a bag filled with fluid the colour of chicken stock, suspending the spindly strands of a strange, excised tumour that once crept along the branches of a nerve path. Near my feet, a pair of red lungs sit in a bucket. There's room in here for twenty-eight bodies, but only nineteen lie here, wrapped like mummies on silver trays, in once wet but now frozen white towels. The fabric is soaked in water and humectants which keep the skin moisturised – with the combined effects of the air-flow in the lab and the amount of chemicals in the embalming fluid, it wouldn't take longer than a week here for a body to dehydrate to the point of leather.

The bodies are sealed inside plastic bags, tied with an ID number on a tag the shape of a fifty-pence piece that matches the one around their neck. Some are resting in an inch of amber-coloured liquid – embalming fluid leaking out of the pores and the injection site. The leak carries on the longer the body stays in the programme; most of the embalming fluid is water, and the human body is not watertight. I ask Terry if this is a messy job and he gives me a look that says, *You have no idea.* He points at the drains in the floor, says the flooring has no seams in it for a reason.

'You smell like it when you go home at night.'

§

Earlier that morning I had arrived on the ninth floor of the Stabile Building to bustle in the front office. Dawn the receptionist told me to take as much Laffy Taffy as I liked from the bowl on the counter, then she was back on the phone, typing notes, the receiver pinned between shoulder and cheek. Shawn was in blue scrubs with his back to me at the computer, and Terry was nowhere to be seen. I filled my pockets with pink, green and yellow candy and looked around the office – piles of paper, inboxes, outboxes, computers, a plant. I was out of stuff to look at and about to read the joke on the back of my candy wrapper when Terry appeared wearing the same blue scrubs as Shawn. It was 9 a.m. and he'd already been here for two and a half hours. He handed a stack of papers to Shawn and said that I'd arrived on a busy morning: they'd had two donor deaths to deal with, and one of them had just pulled into the car park. Shawn is out of his seat and on the case: tall, thin, with intense eyes and a reassuring smile that cracks his face in half. Donate your body to the anatomy school at the Mayo Clinic and these are the guys who look after your corpse.

There's not much else here in Rochester, Minnesota, apart from the clinic. In 1883, three decades after the town was founded, a tornado tore the place apart, leaving thirty-seven dead and two hundred injured. There were no hospitals in the immediate area, just a small practice run by Dr William Mayo. Aided by his two sons – who were practising eye surgery on a sheep's head in a slaughterhouse shortly before the storm hit – he treated the wounded in homes, offices, hotels, even a dance hall, before asking Mother Alfred, of the Sisters of Saint Francis, to use her empty convent as a temporary hospital. It was her idea to raise funds and open a permanent one in a cornfield. She said she'd had a vision from God that it would become world-renowned for its medical arts.

Look at the map and the city looks like it grew around the hospital, with everything feeding back to that shining, iconic facility. Hotels of decreasing appeal spread out from the centre, banners stretched across the fronts of far-flung motels promising free shuttles to the clinic but explicitly no free cable. Other hotels dotted between the high-rise hospital buildings connect doctor and patient by subterranean wheelchair-friendly tunnels carpeted in the kind of technicolour design you'd either want to avoid or seek out while high. In the white, Midwestern winter, nobody has to step outside unless they're leaving town or have run out of restaurants – the tunnels stretch for miles, with overlit gift shops along the way selling 'Get Well' balloons and stuffed bears clutching red love hearts. Antique dealers rack decorative rifles in their windows beside oil paintings of fruit bowls and English hunting dogs, preying on the desire for distraction from what is, if not imminent death, at least something so medically complicated they had to come to one of the world's most respected and experimental medical destinations to try and cure it. They have treated the Dalai Lama for prostate cancer, former President Ronald Reagan underwent brain surgery here, and the comedian Richard Pryor, who was treated for multiple sclerosis, said at a later gig at the Comedy Store, 'You know this shit is bad when you gotta go to the fucking North Pole to find out what's wrong with you.' According to the leaflets piled around the hotel lobby, the Mayo is 'a place for hope where there is no hope'. I have never seen a breakfast buffet crowd lower in spirit.

Terry started here at the Mayo after years of working as a funeral director in this same town. It's an unusual environment for a funeral director – people come here from all over the world to receive treatment, which doesn't always work, and if they die, those bodies need to be returned home. Instead of organising ceremonies and having the connection to families that Poppy does, he was mostly preparing bodies for transport and sending them elsewhere. It was a lot of physical work, and he got burned out on the night calls in particular – death has no consideration for the living's business hours – so when a position opened up here in the clinic twenty-one years ago, he happily bailed.

Now as the director of anatomical services, the state-of-the-art anatomy lab is under Terry's control: he signs you up while you're alive, receives your body when you die, preserves you and files you away in a freezer. In most other academic institutions cadavers are sent to different labs across campus, some pushed across roads on metal gurneys in the dark of early morning, but here, if students and doctors want to work on a body, they come to where the bodies are. They come to Terry.

I found Terry through an ex-colleague of his, Dean Fisher, who I had interviewed the previous year for a *WIRED* magazine article about a new, more environmentally sound method of cremating bodies with super-heated water and lye instead of fire. The process – known as alkaline hydrolysis – was only commercially legal in a dozen or so US states at the time, and Fisher had a machine at the UCLA campus, where he was doing the same job as Terry, and where the machine was used (non-commercially) for the disposal of medical cadavers. When I asked if he could show me how the donated body department worked, he put me in touch with Terry instead – his old college classmate, his fishing pal, his 'brother from another mother'. Fisher said they had worked at the Mayo Clinic together for years and there was more to see there. It was Fisher who had given Terry the job and saved him from the night shifts.

Terry takes me into one of the empty classrooms where an antique wired skeleton – once belonging (externally, not internally) to prominent endocrinologist and Mayo co-founder, Dr Henry Plummer – dangles from a hook by the whiteboard. 'We get a lot of misdirected calls from people who want to donate organs, or they want to donate money,' he says, dragging a couple of chairs over to a desk. 'But we want all of you! We want something more valuable than your money.'

He sits down and slides a letter and contract in front of me. It's the one he sends to all of the prospective donors – who could be patients here, or have family being treated here, or have nothing at all to do with the clinic in life – pre-signed by himself. 'It is my desire to make my body or portion thereof available to further the advancement of medical education and research,' it begins. On the back there are reasons for possible refusal of this gift: 'communicable diseases that pose risk to students and staff, obesity, extreme emaciation, bodies that have been autopsied, mutilated, decomposed, or, for some other reason, are determined to be un-acceptable for anatomical donation.'

'Are people ever offended when you reject a body?' I ask, scanning the list of entry requirements, checking if I'd make the cut.

'Oh yeah, they're on the phone dropping F-bombs! Mostly it's because they didn't read that far into the information. It used to be seven or eight pages, so we've tried to condense it. But the vast majority fit our criteria. Usually the ones that are a hundred years old are in a lot better shape than the ones that are thirty, forty, fifty, sixty – because if they died that young there are some significant issues. You don't live to a hundred by accident.'

He explains that the main thing is that donors have their anatomy intact: once organs are missing, through partial dona-tion or autopsy, students can't learn how everything connects, how the heart relates to the lung, how the arterial system relates to the brain. If you're too fat, they can't find your organs among the adipose (a thick grease that is the colour of butter and just as easy to grip) in the time they're given to complete their modules, and the tables in the lab aren't large enough to accommodate some people. If you're emaciated, there's not much muscle to see and identify, so there's no educational point cutting you open – your bicep might be nothing but a thin strand. 'We don't go off BMI, because it's nonsense,' he says. 'It says I'm obese, but I'd take my body. We look at their age, their activity. A 160-pound female who's been in a wheelchair for years versus a 160-pound female who's been active is gonna be two different bodies, from our perspective.'

There's also the edema (fluid) that pools in swollen extrem-ities after chronic heart failure that makes things more difficult. The goal here is to study textbook anatomy, how the body works and functions. Until students have a grasp of what it should look like when everything's fine, they don't have a baseline to address abnormalities. There's a bit at the end saying that once the clinic accepts a body, you cannot visit it or take it back. He thanks you at

the bottom for considering this most precious gift and signs his
name in blue biro.

This isn't all stated as plainly on the contract as Terry lays it
out for me now, sitting in this empty classroom with his hands
clasped in his lap. But if you had questions before signing, Terry
is not the kind of guy to euphemise facts and bubble-wrap your
feelings: he'll tell you anything you want to know and some
things you don't. If he's anything like he is with me today, he'll
be laughing all the way through, the kind of laughter that sits just
before the tip into hysterics. He is not the first person I've met in
the death industry to make me believe you require a natural level
of cheer high enough that the dip, when it comes, doesn't scrape
the bottom of your heart.

§

Read the history of anatomy and scientific enlightenment and the
names of doctors are lit up like saints and gods. But the history
of medicine is built on a bed of corpses – most with no names
recorded at all.

Academics knew that to further understand the workings of
the human body, and in turn save future lives, they needed dead
bodies to take apart and figure out how they worked. Dissecting
a pig could only tell you so much about a human. They could
learn more from the quiet, inanimate dead than the screaming,
conscious patient, and if they knew what they were doing, fewer
people would die on the table. But there was no system for a
person to will their body to science. There was no contract. There
was no Terry.

The shift from carrying out dissections on animals to the human
dead was a focus of political, societal and religious tension, all of
which is discussed at length in Ruth Richardson's excellent book
Death, Dissection and the Destitute. Initially, it had been ruled by James IV
in 1506 that the Edinburgh Guild of Surgeons and Barbers could
have access to certain executed criminals for dissection. England
then followed in 1540, when Henry VIII granted anatomists an
annual right to the bodies of four hanged felons, and later six,

when Charles II – a patron of the sciences – gave them a further two. Dissection became recognised by law as a punishment, added to the array of existing punishments – a special fate worse than death, to be carried out publicly, described as 'further Terror and a peculiar Mark of Infamy'. It was an alternative to being hanged, drawn and quartered – where body parts were hoisted on spikes throughout the city, the ultimate punishment in a religious society where bodies were supposed to remain whole in preparation for the resurrection. Some prisoners who had been sentenced to death but not dissection would – prior to their execution – barter their own corpses with agents of surgeons so they could buy fancy outfits to die in. They were the first, purely by shitty circumstance, to opt in to body donation.

The problem was there weren't enough bodies. Anatomists did what they felt they needed to do: William Harvey, whose published work in 1628 proved the circulation of blood, dissected his own father and sister. Others robbed fresh graves in the night, or their pupils did. The corpse, because of its scarcity, became a commodity, and to make up for the shortfall in supply from the gallows, the bodysnatching industry was created. 'Resurrectionists' would dig up the recently dead – most often the mass graves of the urban poor – and deliver them to the anatomy schools in exchange for cash. By the 1720s – a hundred years after William Harvey dissected his family to discover the path of blood – stealing bodies from London graveyards was, if not exactly common, at least widespread enough that it was verging on being so. The two leading anatomists of their generation, William Hunter and his younger brother John, worked constantly on the bodies of humans and animals, a method that would have been impossible with the number of corpses provided by the hangman. In the 1750s, when John Hunter was responsible for sourcing bodies for his older brother's anatomy school, he bought them from resurrectionists or dug them up himself. It was during this period that he filled his famous museum, the Hunterian, with medical marvels and mutations. It still stands by Lincoln's Inn Fields in London, with disembodied hearts and tiny babies staring out of the same chemical that preserves two-headed lizards and a lion's toes. I have stood there in front of the cabinets and stared back.

By the time Mary Shelley was born in 1797, bodysnatching was rife, and it was no secret, either; when she was a young adult, various contraptions, like iron cages to hold coffins, were being sold specifically to thwart the resurrectionists. Bodies were stolen from the churchyard where her mother Mary Wollstonecraft was buried, where the story goes that her father had taught her to write her name by tracing over the carved letters on her mother's headstone. Ultimately, it fed into her work: none of the bodies that became the monster in Frankenstein had signed a contract to be there – he is nameless, a product, a belonging – while the real monster was the scientist, who was so gripped by the idea of his own creation that he disregarded what was right.

Things reached a head in 1828 when Burke and Hare made themselves infamous in Edinburgh for skipping the exhumation and going straight to murder, with payment on delivery. Burke was executed for his sixteen suffocations and sentenced to dissection as an ironic post-mortem punishment. His skeleton still stands in the anatomical museum in the University of Edinburgh with a paper sign pinned to his rib: (IRISH MALE) The skeleton of WILLIAM BURKE, THE NOTORIOUS MURDERER. Some 332 miles south, a piece of his brain sits at the bottom of a jar in the Wellcome Collection in London, pale and shrunken. When I saw it in an exhibition in 2012, it was placed on the same shelf as a slice of Einstein's brain. Genius or villain, the mind as matter looks much the same.

Something had to be done to kill the industry of bodysnatching while continuing to feed the machine of science and education. So came the Anatomy Act of 1832, which stipulated that surgeons could take the unclaimed dead from prisons, poorhouses, asylums and hospitals – thereby equating 'poor' with 'felon', which led to a whole other world of social turmoil. But the anatomists got their bodies, regardless of the dead's wishes, and the poor had something new to add to their list of fears.

One of the first people to voluntarily donate their body to science was the English philosopher Jeremy Bentham, whose severed head we were celebrating 186 years after all life had left it. When he died in 1832, two months before the Anatomy Act was passed, he had stipulated in his will that he wished to be publicly dissected by Dr Southwood Smith, who had previously written about how burial was a waste of bodies that could be better used in teaching. Bentham too wanted to demonstrate the usefulness of the corpse to the living – and the comparative uselessness of burying a tool of scientific study for the worms to eat – and light the way for a movement that would benefit the world. On a pamphlet handed out at the dissection was a line from his will about his decision: 'This my will and special request I make, not out of affectation of singularity, but to the intent and with the desire that mankind may reap some small benefit in and by my decease, having hitherto had small opportunities to contribute thereto while living.'

Despite his efforts, anatomical donation wouldn't catch on for another hundred years or so. Ruth Richardson speculates in her book that since the rise in bequests coincides with an increased cremation rate, perhaps the spiritual associations of the corpse had changed in the post-war period: cremation would render a corpse no longer whole for the resurrection, as would dissection.

Today's UK medical cadavers are now exclusively the bodies of those who have donated them, which isn't true of everywhere in the world: most countries in Africa and Asia study unclaimed bodies, while Europe, South America and North America are a mix of unclaimed and donated. There is, occasionally, a strange blend of the old world and the new – where someone has opted in, but perhaps not to the extent the future has taken it. Currently, a virtual autopsy table called the Anatomage is available for use in medical training: it's a touchscreen tablet the size of a real autopsy table, programmed with layers and layers of images, each a 1mm 'slice' of the body, together creating a three-dimensional whole that students can look inside without actually touching a real person. Two of the four bodies, one male and one female, were part of the Visible Human Project – a project run by the US National Library of

Medicine in the mid-nineties – who made the images by freezing the body, then grinding a 1mm layer off each time a new photograph was taken. At a conference in Manchester, I got to try out the table while the hovering sales representative explained its functionality. I stooped there in the small crowd, poking, prodding, turning the body, zooming in on organs most will likely never see in real life, in full, detailed colour. The one I was looking at was an executed murderer from Texas, Joseph Paul Jernigan, who agreed to donate his body to science, though the ethics of its current use have been questioned. He would have been unaware of the availability of the images: an interactive autopsy table had not yet been invented when he was killed by lethal injection in 1993.

Last year, 236 people who signed Terry's contract died and made their donation, willing their body to a fate once reserved for criminals. Twenty years ago that number topped out at fifty. Popularity is growing, and currently around 700 new donors sign up every year. Considering that bodies are willed directly to the Mayo (instead of a central body-brokering organisation that divides them among various facilities, which is how many other donation programmes work), I ask Terry why this place would receive so many. It feels so deliberate. Their numbers are higher than UCLA, which has a similar direct-donation programme, and has averaged 168 bodies a year over the last ten; but California has a population of nearly 40 million, with 4 million in Los Angeles alone. In Minnesota, there's just over 5 million people spread out over the state, which in terms of landmass is not far off the entirety of England. Driving to Rochester from the main airport in Minneapolis, you're on flat, endless roads. You're in cornfield country. There's nobody but you and some dairy cows.

'A lot of it comes from the good care they had when they were a patient here; they want to give something back,' he says. 'They're training the next generation that's going to provide good care to their next generation. Coming from the funeral director's side, we bury or cremate the bodies – that's the end of their story. Their contribution to society ends. Here, it continues.'

What more can you give back than your whole self?

§

When Terry was eighteen, he was enlisted in the Navy, mainly working in the Intensive Care Unit at a large Naval hospital in Virginia, where he drew blood as part of the crash team. It was the tail end of the Vietnam War, and there were guys his own age coming in to be treated. It was the first time Terry had been around the dying, and the deaths were hard to emotionally compute – young men admitted for what appeared to be nothing more exotic than asthma would leave in a body bag. 'There were babies in the neonatal department that had a lot of problems, and that was easier to take than someone who was talking to me last week, joking around like a normal person you'd meet on the street, and then watching him die.' Terry would escort the deceased patients to the morgue, and it was there he met his first funeral directors. He wasn't sure what he wanted to do as a career, and there they were, taking care of people past the point where he was able.

William Hunter, the older anatomist brother, said in an introductory lecture to students that 'anatomy is the very basis of surgery … it informs the head, gives dexterity to the hand, and familiarises the heart with a sort of necessary inhumanity.' In other words, clinical detachment is necessary for this system to work. Medicine would not have advanced as much as it has if it were not for the dead in the anatomy rooms. We needed to learn about ourselves to save ourselves. But while clinical detachment is a necessity, Terry is keen to get across the fact that respect for the dead is what rules this hospital kingdom. Someone untrained in the funeral industry might run this programme very differently, but for him the science never fully separates the body from the person they were. 'The needs of the patient come first, and we hold that true here even though they're deceased. We treat them like a patient, we protect their medical records, their name, their privacy, their confidentiality,' he says. 'We maintain that like they are alive.'

He spends a lot of time trying to get this through to the students, who see a divide between themselves and the body in front of them. 'Maybe it helps them emotionally, to pretend death didn't happen,' he says. 'Maybe it gives them some security to think about them as more of an inanimate object, because they're young, they haven't seen much of death. So they kind of minimise the gift, or minimise the person to an object that they can make fun of. I don't think it's purposeful, I think it's a coping mechanism.' For the students, this is usually their first sight of a dead body, and fainting is not uncommon. Terry says he's picked most of them up off the floor. 'I've caught people in the hallways, or here in the classroom – they just turn into a noodle, and they slide off the chairs.'

The divide is something I can empathise with, but for a different reason. I think back to the virtual autopsy table I saw at the conference in Manchester and how, surrounded by people excited by a new machine, I immediately selected the option to look at the rudest parts. I didn't want to see his lungs, I wanted to see the dead man's dick – everybody did. There was a disconnect: even though we were being told that these were images of a real person, the novelty of the touchscreen worked as a barrier. These were just photographs, this was like a game. There was no personality to piece together like I did with Adam in the mortuary; death did not feel tangible through the glass. There was no reverence: the man was naked, devoid of personality, whatever it is that makes us more than pure anatomy. But this is why Terry keeps the nail polish, the tattoos – he keeps just enough to serve as a reminder that this was a living, breathing person. In some programmes, he also gives out their cause of death, age, occupation. If I were a medical student, I doubt that I could ever feel that same connection to a body through a screen, to feel what Terry says is essential to learn not just the mechanics but the meaning of the job you're studying for. The experience has been hollowed out: the most important person isn't there, so death isn't either. You would need to, like I did in that sunlit mortuary, touch them. Be in their presence, even if it overwhelmed you, initially, to the point of fainting. They might not feel what I did instantly with Adam, but it would come. Terry makes sure of it.

'Our donors are the best people in the world,' he says, with genuine wonder. 'It's a very, very personal gift, giving someone your body. Can you think of anything more personal or private? Some of the eighty- or ninety-year-olds – they lived through mini-skirts and all that, this very conservative generation. To allow someone to dissect and go through every bit of their body? It's quite a sacrifice, to gift someone something that they've protected, and been conservative with, all their lives.'

§

Terry goes to check what's going on in the lab and returns in a white lab coat, the coast apparently all clear of I'm not exactly sure what. We walk down the hall past framed photos of all the staff. Everyone is smiling big American smiles.

The anatomy laboratory is brightly lit and Terry asks me what it smells like – he can't tell any more. 'The dentist?' I say. He laughs. 'I'm worried about your dentist.' A ventilation system pushes the heavy carcinogenic gas used in the embalming of bodies (the in-jectable preservative fluid 'formalin' is formaldehyde gas saturated with methyl alcohol so it becomes liquid, but evaporation turns it gaseous again) towards the bottom of the room and pumps in oxygen from above, a constantly moving cycle of air, so that the preservatives in the bodies don't negatively affect the health of those working on them, and there's less likelihood of the nausea that sent my fellow students in high school fleeing from their dissected toad. He points at the vents in the ceiling and the others near the floor, which is sealed to allow water from arthroscopic surgery – a kind of keyhole surgery with a camera – to pour down. The water is needed for the clarity of the image the camera captures, he tells me: it's like wearing a scuba mask on the beach versus wearing it underwater. He pushes heavy plastic work tables around with ease to show that they move on wheels. Anglepoise lamps hang from the ceiling every couple of feet. There are wires and plugs and sockets, computer monitors and television screens, and on the far right of the room there are glass-fronted cabinets filled with anatomy books and bizarre objects. He opens one and points at something large and grey. 'You know regular household latex that sits in the cracks in your walls?' He picks up what looks like sun-faded coral intricately carved from styrofoam. Terry had poured latex into a pair of inflated lungs and submerged the whole thing in bleach, and when the tissue dissolved it left him with these: a 3D roadmap for oxygen, feather-light human lungs.

From a high shelf he pulls down a huge Tupperware container of artefacts found inside cadavers over the years, kept to show the students earlier versions of what they may be learning to install. A Harrington rod that once fused a spine, a heart bypass valve, a grape-sized testicular implant that bounces once as he chucks it back in the box. A plastic patella. A pacemaker. A bone screw. An antique breast implant. Aortic mesh. Stents that propped open the chambers of hearts. These are the things we ordinarily bury with our dead. Even greener, natural burial grounds are littered with the metal of factory-made knees.

Now he's opening drawers and lifting things up into the light, making them worse by naming them: bone saws, delicate needle-eye-sized skin hooks for plastic surgery, hip retractors, rib shears, chest spreaders. Curettes for scraping, scissors with blades that bend at all kinds of angles to get into the most difficult-to-reach areas. Scalpels, mallets, chisels and forceps. 'It's *Tool Time* goes to college, you know?' He holds up something that looks truly evil, like a metal snake with a serrated mouth, and says, 'This thing oscillates back and forth and chews up the tissue, then it sucks it out.' Small bits of shining steel are glinting in their neat dividers, everything put away in its labelled drawer. 'These are about a grand apiece!' he says, obviously thrilled to show off the collection.

On the bench are sutures, tape, paper towels, skin staplers. There are gloves and aprons of all sizes, a sink, an autoclave – even though there's no risk of infection from one patient to the next, the implements are kept surgery-spotless. There are boxes of eye protectors, full face shields, partial face shields, knee-high shoe covers for the wet lab. Now he's pulling out the equipment they'll be using in a hip-replacement class this afternoon: the 'reamers' that clear out the marrow before insertion of a rod or nail, various hammers, the ball joints in green, blue and pink plastic. He shows me what looks like a golf-ball-sized cheese grater and tells me that this is what they use to make space in the socket for the joint. He twists it in the air, miming the motion of grating. Parts of me begin to ache.

'I don't faint around dead bodies,' I say, in case my face is about to ruin my chances of seeing the whole of the lab. 'But, uh, bone graters might be beyond my limit.' He chuckles again and points across the room. 'Well, those are carts full of brains.'

He invites me to open a tub of my choosing. We peer in at the blue-veined grey slices, cut uniformly like a loaf of bread. In fact, that's the lab terminology: this brain has been 'breadloafed' along the axial plane. 'Do you ever look at that and think about how this chunk controlled a whole person?' I ask, the slices jostling against each other in the preservative.

'The whole body is a miracle. And looking at how the brain contributes it's ... it's just mind-boggling. So these are the stainless operating tables that I talked about, the ones that open like clams—'

As Terry talks about the Wi-Fi connection and the various upgrades made over the years, my eyes wander across the room and I see a body lying on a table. It's covered in a white sheet, some brownish-red stains here and there. Two feet stick out: old and gnarly, the toenails extend a centimetre beyond the toe it-self. It's the body of a man, but the feet are shaped like he's been shoehorning them into the pointiest of uncomfortable stilettos. He has no head. He's patiently waiting for his new hip.

§

'Legs are in the back, heads and uppers on the sides,' Terry says, stepping out so I can go in on my own, a slim walkway between shelving so high you'd require a ladder to reach the top level. This is the freezer where the fresh tissue is kept; unlike those in the cool room, there is no preservative in these bodies. 'We want to try to create a model that's close to what the user will see in their patient, minus the pulse and breathing,' he explains from the doorway. Not only does embalming limit the flexibility of the tissue, the chemicals tend to bleach it of its colour; students approaching a live body for the first time, having only operated on an embalmed one, would have learned their way on a faded map. 'We try to recreate that surgical environment to get them as close as they can be to real patient care. This is the spot to make their mistakes.'

There are no whole bodies here, just pieces of what Terry estimates to be about 130 donors. Stand in a cemetery surrounded by thousands of bodies and you don't think about the difference six feet of earth makes; here the visual crowd is what staggers. Hundreds of bags of shapes line the walls. I can see fingers and feet, and what could be footballs were it not for the noses pressed against the plastic. One bagged head has a doctor's name written on it in permanent blue marker – reserved for later use. On the floor there's a whole leg with a hip joint attached, its bare foot poking out from the towel. The green bags denote 'finished' pieces – these body parts are ready to be cremated, and are just waiting here for the rest of the person to turn up, all identified by a unique number. When they all get here, Terry will lay the pieces out and rebuild a human, but he won't stitch them together: the flesh is too frozen to take a needle and thread, and if they thawed they would leak. They'll be cremated in full, and get their name and identity back. 'That's a promise that we hold very, very strong to our families. We don't lose anything.'

'Some people might view this as disrespectful,' he says, motioning past me into the depths of the freezer. 'To me it would be disrespectful to have tissue go to waste.'

I paused there in the cold, looking down at these pieces of people, patches of crystalline frost misting up the plastic. I tried to work out what it was I was feeling. When I first contacted Terry, I predicted this scene would be more shocking to the senses, that despite years of staring into jars at pathology museums, this would be different and likely harder to look at. These would not be the pale specimens from long ago – these would be recent, fleshy, dis-tinctly human, and somewhere in a computer system they would have names. Someone would still be grieving for them. But there was a disconnect, not just physically with the bags and towels, but emotionally: none of these items corresponded to people as I recognise them. The only thing that got me were the hands, with their perfectly polished nails or roughly bitten ones – that student was right. Hands retain a personality even after they are severed. They are things that people held, they're the thing we're supposed to know the back of better than anything. On a shelf beside me were arms half wrapped in small towels, twisted into clear bags, separated from the body just below the shoulder. Here were hands paused mid-sentence in sign language, caught in a moment of effusive gesticulation, here they were frozen in time – collected gestures removed from body and context, orphaned frames of a Muybridge set. Bare hands in bags have more personality than entire bodies.

But I felt almost nothing, or at least none of what I had expected. There was no shock, fear or repulsion in the freezer of decapitated heads: it was pure science and *Futurama*. I had felt the loss of thirteen lives in Poppy's mortuary, but though here there were ten times that in pieces in front of me, there was a strange emotional silence.

Charles Byrne, the seven-foot-seven Irish Giant, knew when his health began to deteriorate in the 1780s that the anatomists were after his body. He did not want to end up in John Hunter's museum of pathological specimens, a freak show preserved in a glass cabinet for centuries, looking down at the tourists in their puffer jackets. So he asked to be buried at sea, and when he died at the age of twenty-two his body was taken to the coast. Most of the pieces of people in the Hunterian Museum are anonymous, bodysnatched. But there Byrne stands: the stolen, named skeleton who never made it to the ocean, whose empty coffin was weighed down with rocks by the bribed undertaker so the pallbearers wouldn't notice. Looking up at his thick bones, you cannot help but feel the emotional weight of them. He did not want to be there.

It hit me, slowly, that everyone in that freezer at that moment, including Terry, and including me, wanted to be there. All of this death, layer upon layer of frozen flesh, bag upon bag of legs and torsos, could drown the life in the room if you let it. The relentless butcher-shop sameness, the cold and the thaw, the filing and the numbering – it could render all of this meaningless or worse. But here the sheer scale of it performed a cosmic trick. Zoom out and take it in all at once: this scene was not shocking or sad, because every single person wanted some good to come from their death, and this was what they chose. Here was a picture of profound generosity and hope, framed by the rubber seal of a heavy-duty silver door.

§

Decapitate the common snapping turtle and the jaw will still clamp, like an amputated lizard's tail will still twist in the grass. Its heart can beat cold blood for hours. Thanks to its strength and hardness of shell, the snapping turtle has no natural predators bar fans of turtle soup, passing cars and bored boys.

It was the mid-1960s, in Florida, when seven-year-old Terry found the remains of a turtle neighbourhood bullies had tormented and abandoned. He returned to the crime scene daily, marvelling at the life remaining in the animated head, the pure reactive nature of muscle biology, the trademark snap that gave the reptile its descriptor. Crouching over it in the sticky heat, he became fascinated with the miracle of a body in life and death, its function and base mechanics. In his memory, it took five days for the decapitated turtle to stop biting the stick.

Terry looks at me like a man who hasn't thought about this in a while. After the snapping turtle he took his Red Ryder BB gun to the Everglades National Park to hunt bobwhite quail, armadillos, raccoons and possums. He'd remove the viscera, always curious about what was on the inside. 'Instead of having Kool-Aid stands, I'd go out and shoot sharks, cut their jaws off and see what they'd been eating. Then I'd sell the jaws on the A1A, the big highway in Florida. And coconuts. I couldn't believe all the old people that were buying coconuts.' All this might sound like the makings of another Jeffrey Dahmer, but an interest in death doesn't always lead down the same path. Terry was looking for the life in the body, the thing that electrified the parts.

Now, using medical equipment on established surgical planes, Terry takes apart the bodies to preserve the structures the students need to study. To partition a shoulder, he will cut along the clavicle, follow the rib cage, and separate the arm with the shoulder blade attached. To get the maximum use out of knees and ankles but reserve the hips for another department, he will leave a third of a femur for the orthopaedic students to observe the hip approach. To take a head off a body, he uses a bone saw to cut through the flesh and disarticulates the vertebrae somewhere above the shoulders, keeping as much of the neck as possible so someone can study the airways.

I ask if any of this bothers him. He laughs and says no, he's seen worse things picking up bodies at crime scenes than anything he could personally do in the prep room. He doesn't know what it is about him that allows him to do this job that others can't, what it is that precludes him from nausea and nightmares and fainting. When he was a funeral director, the coroner in Rochester didn't have a removal team, so Terry was regularly asked to do it. While he methodically went about picking up pieces of bodies in the aftermath of a car explosion that melted the seats to springs, colleagues retched in front of local news cameras. Others coated their nostrils in Vicks and stood aside while Terry bagged up a suicide that had lain dead in a squat for weeks, beside a handgun wrapped in magazines to muffle the noise. He's collected people whose pets have eaten their faces off, and all of it has been fine. I keep asking how he stands it, how he does it, and he keeps chuckling. He doesn't know. I let the question hang a little longer.

'Well, I had to take a friend's head off. That was...' He trails off. 'There's still not a day in my career that I don't remove somebody's head or arm, that I wonder how I got this job. How did I end up here?'

The friend was a colleague at the Mayo who had willed his body to the programme. Terry reasoned with himself that the guy knew what he was signing up for and who was going to be doing it, so he was carrying out his wishes. 'I've accepted quite a few donors in my years here that I've known, and it changes it. I still detach myself and keep my promise that we're gonna do everything we can do to honour their gift, but there's always a personal side of things. But you have to just go on. I'm sure the physicians and healthcare providers, if their friends or family come in, it changes things for them too. It's a little more pressure, you still want to do a good job, but you're gonna do everything the same for the other patient you don't know. But it changes the emotional approach to it.'

Sometimes you have to keep watch on your own heart, though: there is now a system in place, an agreement with a neighbouring university in Minneapolis, whereby they can swap bodies if they're too close to the staff or students.

'Did you do anything differently for your friend?' I ask. 'Did you cover his face?'

'Nope. I just went to work and tried to squash my emotions and just do my normal, good job to fulfil their wish of participating.'

I wonder, though, if it's a learned habit; even for a funeral director, a freezer full of decapitated heads is an unusual sight. So I ask if this was a shock on his first day, when they had thirteen heads lined up across two tables for courses in thyroplasty and rhinoplasty. 'I didn't run away,' he says. 'I just thought, *Well, that's weird*.' He believes that working in funeral homes probably had more emotional downsides: funeral homes, unlike the Mayo's anatomy department, deal with the bodies of children – something he has always found particularly hard to process. 'You're dealing with grief all the time. I deal with that a little bit in this role, but it also gives the family a lot of hope and optimism, something positive coming out of a really bad situation.' He thinks about it a little longer, searching for something else to explain why the heads don't faze him. 'No, I'm comfortable as heck!' he says, coming up with nothing. 'Doesn't bother me at all. If we just cut the heads off without seeing the benefit, I might have bigger issues.'

Terry is sixty-two, and in two years he'll be retiring, though he seems like the kind of person who will always be two years away from retiring. But he hasn't planned his life around it – he knows there's a chance a person won't make it to retiring age. He also knows that the human jaw does not live on like a snapping turtle, but a body can keep on giving once the life in it has gone: it can help the living in more ways than offering up a warm liver in the last moments on a hospital bed. It's impossible to quantify the number of errors prevented or successes they've achieved in this lab, because it's all part of training young doctors – but there is a very direct line from the dead in his freezers to the living on the street.

Once or twice a month a doctor will ask for his help. There was the doctor who perfected his tool to cure carpal tunnel syndrome on the wrists of the dead. Then there was the doctor who came to him with the problem of a tumour so complex and potentially fatal that surgeons worldwide had refused to touch it; it started at the neck and wrapped its way down around the patient's spinal column like the red stripe on a barber's pole, stopping below the chest. A multidisciplinary team would need to be involved with the different stages of removing this twisted mass – rolling through the surgical specialities as they moved further down the spine, front to back, front to back, rotating the man like a rotisserie chicken – so they practised in Terry's lab, arriving at 10 p.m. after work, leaving at dawn, turning the bodies of the dead, working out their plan. The patient survived.

Then there was the face transplant. I had already heard about it: the fifty-six-hour marathon surgery was so successful it made international news. The thirty-two-year-old patient, Andy Sandness from Wyoming – a state in the heart of the American male suicide epidemic – destroyed most of his face with a self-inflicted gunshot wound to the chin at twenty-one. A decade later, Calen Ross shot himself and died in south-western Minnesota. Their ages, blood type, skin colour and facial structure were a near-perfect match. The doctors had spent three years waiting for the right donor, practising. To prepare for the operation, the surgeons, nurses, surgical technicians and anaesthetists spent fifty weekends in Terry's lab, divided into two small rooms to replicate the cramped operating room. They studied every branch of nerves and what they did for the face; they took pictures and videos, and practised joining them up. Every time they came in, they worked on two different heads. They swapped 100 faces. The donors don't leave here in one piece, but Terry makes sure they leave with the right ones. So when the surgeons were done, he would stay behind and swap the faces back. No one would ever have known if he hadn't. There is no bone in the facial flesh that would end up in the wrong urn after the cremation. He did it because it was the right thing to do, in much the same way that he, as a funeral director, always made sure everyone was buried in outfits complete with underwear and socks, even if their family had forgotten to add them to the shopping bag of clothes. Sure, no one would know if he didn't do it – but he would.

It's this part of the work that keeps him going through the bone saws and the decapitations: the scientific advancement, the possibilities, the fundamental good that is intrinsic in the work that is carried out here. He has an assistant who also cuts up the bodies, and Terry encourages him to occasionally come out of the freezer to see the students, to see what his work leads to; without the science and the hope, Terry knows the environment could be a sad one to work in. But his face lights up when he talks about his involvement in the continuing lives of the living, as hidden in the cold backroom as he may be.

§

A podiatrist, failing spectacularly at small talk at a party, once told me that everyone wants to keep their foot in a jar. She mostly worked with returned veterans who – through neglect or diabetes, usually both – had let their feet rot. She said nobody wants to lose their foot no matter what state it's in, that people would rather keep it rotting on the end of their leg and have it kill them than have it taken away. If they concede the foot is a lost cause, they ask if they can keep it. People don't want to let pieces of themselves go.

I think of these men looking up from their wheelchairs, desperately pleading to keep their putrid feet in jars, as Terry slows the body collection van to a stop in Oakwood Cemetery. He's out of his scrubs now. In his orange plaid Harley-Davidson shirt, blue jeans and brown boots he looks more like he should be leaning on his 1800cc Ultra Classic outside a dive bar, not driving a white Dodge van through a neat graveyard in rural Minnesota. He jokes that I'm the only passenger he's ever had sit up front.

He winds down the window and points at the grey granite memorial that has been erected for every donor that ever came through the Mayo Clinic, a vault for the people who gave away their entire bodies knowing no specifics about what it would go through or by whose scalpel they would be taken unskilfully apart. Engraved into the front of the monument are these words:

> DEDICATED TO THE INDIVIDUALS
> WHO HAVE DONATED THEIR
> BODIES TO MAYO FOUNDATION
> FOR ANATOMICAL STUDY
> SO THAT OTHERS MIGHT LIVE.

Terry comes here regularly to keep an eye on the damp inside the vault, to trim the grass around the stone, and every year he comes to add more ashes. He tends this grave for the thousands of people he never knew while they were alive, but whose bodies he looked after until they were cremated, in pieces, a year after they died.

Not everybody is here: if the families want the ashes back, they collect them at an annual service called the Convocation of Thanks, where they go from anonymised body to person again. On black plastic urns they get their names back, and their donor serial number too – a double life in one body. The ceremony gives thanks to donors but also some kind of conclusion to families – these people haven't had their funeral yet. This year's ceremony is happening tomorrow, and Terry tells me to get there early if I want to secure a seat. They're expecting hundreds.

The next day a crowd is funnelled through a door in the side of the building and directed into a huge auditorium. Medical students read poems at the podium, ones they have written themselves, then return to their seat, not knowing if the person beside them is the brother, son, daughter, wife of the person they dissected. Every poem talks about the basic things they will never know about these people, despite knowing the intricacies of their literal heart. Did they tap their fingers on the steering wheel at stoplights? Did they eat peanut butter out of the jar? In the audience, there are old men in braces, young men wearing cowboy boots and boleros, farmers looking uncomfortable in suits. Wearing blue eyeshadow like 1960s time capsules, hunched women in the line to the bathroom gush about how many girls are in the group photos of young orthopaedic surgeons. The room is buzzing.

Hundreds of donor names are listed on a giant screen and read out one by one by a pair of trainee surgeons, but whoever it was that taught them, personally, the workings of the human body, goes by anonymously in the roll call. A weirdly high number of them are called Kermit. A handsome older man sitting next to me in his suit and yellow tie leans over and tells me quietly but proudly as her name comes up, 'Selma was my mother – 105 and a half!' She was widowed for four decades and won exercise competitions at the nursing home before donating the body she had looked after so carefully – the body that grew this man from an egg she was born with.

Later, around an emptying buffet, people politely wait for the right time to ask Terry for their person back. He's in a dark suit now, and speaks to the families with a quiet and gentle reverence, as if he were by a graveside. Some try their luck and ask if the students ever found anything abnormal inside their father. *How big was the cancer in the end? Do you think it's genetic?* The plates of food congeal. The man in the yellow tie collects his mother. Outside in the Minnesota sunlight, on Cinco de Mayo, old people in wheelchairs wait for ramps to unfold from taxis, boxes of bone dust in their laps.

Click Your Fingers and They Turn to Stone

Nick Reynolds spent his childhood on the run in Mexico with his father, the infamous Great Train Robbery mastermind Bruce Reynolds, and now lives not far from me in London – in a flat on the second floor, on a hill so high there are no buildings obscuring the sky outside the window, nothing between him and the sun but atmosphere. It's a thin warren crammed with art, tour lanyards and bronze heads. I lean against the doorframe in the kitchen while Nick walks from room to room talking, looking for things, telling me he's been flat out for days, that he has to be on a tour bus at eight in the morning, that he can't find the thing he saved to show me – a thank-you letter from a client. As he makes me a mug of tea, he motions past the chaos of dishes, chisels and teabags towards a white plaster face on the bench by the window. He stops working just after sunset, he says, because working is pointless once the light has gone. It's dark outside now, and the details of the man's features are lost in the stark flood of the kitchen bulb. It's clearly a face, and a handsome one, but without that visible detail it would be hard to remember it. 'A suicide,' he says. 'He threw himself off Beachy Head. Took a running jump too, by all accounts.' Near the plaster head, which Nick says he had to patch up in post-production – his jaw was out of line, there were inch-deep dents in his skull from the fall – there is a plaster hand and a plaster foot. Nick doesn't know why someone would want pieces of a man who could have landed in pieces. He tends not to ask why anyone wants the things he makes.

Death masks, throughout history, have had many lives. They have been the realm of kings and pharaohs, used in the making of effigies so that dead royalty could travel their land and people could pay their final respects to an imperishable leader, no matter how long the trip. They were an artist's reference tool before the invention of photography, for use in the making of portraits, and largely discarded afterwards – the artist's rendering deemed more important and befitting than a three-dimensional print straight from the person's face. Death masks were also cast of unknown dead in the hopes of one day identifying them. One of them, taken of a young woman pulled from the Seine in the early 1800s, is now the most kissed face in the world, appearing on the very first CPR training doll, Resusci Anne, in 1960. Albert Camus, who kept a copy of the mask, called her the drowned Mona Lisa. The surrealists made her their static, silent muse. Maybe you've met her. Maybe you've saved a life because you did.

Earlier that day, I had been flipping through a book called *Undying Faces* by Ernst Benkard. Published (in English) in 1929, it's a collection of death masks ranging from the fourteenth century up to the twentieth. Friedrich Nietzsche is here, Leo Tolstoy, Victor Hugo, Mahler, Beethoven. Famous people, rich people, political leaders. All of these dead faces, preserved in plaster, moments, days or weeks after they breathed their last. But why make a death mask now? If you want to preserve an image, why not just take a photograph? Why take a cast of a dead person's face when so many people cannot bear to look at the dead body at all? It had been months since I'd visited the Mayo Clinic and I kept replaying one scene in my mind: Terry staying behind, swapping back the faces of the medical cadavers. What is in a face?

I've come here to ask Nick, who has been casting the faces of the dead for over twenty years, and is the only person doing it (commercially, anyway) in the UK. I had seen his work on headstones in Highgate Cemetery, near where I live: the bronze head of Malcolm McLaren sits above the sandblasted quote, 'Better a spectacular failure, than a benign success'. I had seen Nick's father too. He's not all that far from the entrance. You can almost see his face if you stick your own through the bars of the fence.

We've moved to the black leather sofa in the lounge, a room filled with more books, more sculpture, more painted canvases, the gathered clutter from a life lived among artists and musicians. There's a book on Johnny Cash on the coffee table; glass-fronted cabinets of objects line the walls. A cast of his father's head looks down on us – taken while he was alive, unlike the death mask that sits on top of his grave – and next to it, another life mask of fellow train robber Ronnie Biggs, who became a rebel folk icon while living for thirty-six years as a fugitive from the British police. Biggs wears a pair of black sunglasses and a black hat, like a shop mannequin. Nick keeps copies of his more famous death masks, but all the masks in this room are of the living. Even so, there's something unnerving about them. I feel watched. 'I've had guests stay with me, and there's not a single dead person in here,' he says, motioning towards them. 'But just *masks* freak people out,' he says. 'Just faces.'

He sits back, rolling a cigarette and nursing a can of San Miguel in his lap. He's fifty-seven, wearing a pink shirt, the top few buttons undone, orange-tinted glasses. He coughs and tells me he mostly earns a living as a harmonica player (he's in the band Alabama 3 – you'll have heard them over the opening credits for *The Sopranos*), and the fact that he smokes as much as he does is like killing the golden goose. 'I must be stupid,' he says, licking the edge of the paper. 'If I don't have lungs I can't play.' His voice is low and gravelly, one that could cut through the noise of a loud bar, through the cumulus nicotine fog, and still be heard. The room fills with clouds so quickly he has to open the window so I can breathe.

'In the old days, death masks were important because they thought they were somehow bottling up part of the essence of the person,' he says, blowing smoke out the window. 'They believed in animism. The Greeks and the Romans believed that through concentration, prayer and incantations, whatever, you could summon up the spirit of the person. They believed that statues would come to life. In their mind they would be a house, a repository for whoever the god was, or the person, and they could summon their spirit into it. And I think the Victorians really believed in that too, somehow: that it was a receptacle because it looked like the person. Benkard, in that book you have, said eloquently that it seems that somehow, during the process, part of the mystery of death seems to slip into the casting, and that's what gives them that otherworldly feel.'

Looking at the faces in the book, and the death masks in real life, I do feel that they do hold a kind of magic. They give you proximity to the dead, without being near them – the dead feel closer than those in the photographs on the touchscreen autopsy table in Manchester. They're a form of immortality; a kind of physical limbo between life and death. A person might be dead for 400 years, and you can still see the wrinkles fan out from their eyes without the intermediary of a painter's brush. Nick says a death mask can create a focal point to talk to somebody, whether you believe in an afterlife or not. He talks to his dad's mask. He says that some clients stick them in a drawer and never open it. Others place them on the pillow beside them while they sleep.

He pulls some of his work down from the shelves. Here's Peter O'Toole's enormous hand cast in black, previously seen holding cigarettes in film stills, or in paparazzi shots slung around the shoulders of friends leaving Soho bars. I place my own hand over it and I'm dwarfed. He died in 2013, and through a trick of time and circumstance just happened to be in the funeral home at the same moment as Biggs. Nick phoned up O'Toole's daughter Kate, whom he knew anyway from his work in the band, and asked her, while standing there between the two dead men, if she would like a death mask of her father. (In a BBC interview years later, Kate O'Toole laughed that it was 'classic O'Toolery' that he would end up in the mortuary drawer beside Biggs.)

In past years, Nick thought that the popularity of death masks was on the rise. Any time he cast the face of somebody famous, there would be a newspaper article and some new flurry of interest. Malcolm McLaren. Soho dandy Sebastian Horsley. O'Toole. He had visions of employing art students in different cities to take the casts for him, as an apprenticeship, and he would make the finished masks here in London. But it never really took off. He casts four or five dead people a year, himself, wheeling home the plaster casts from the mortuary in his little wheelie suitcase. They are a strange minority, these people who employ him. There are the families of the rich and famous, who have them done as a tradition – the British Conservative politician Jacob Rees-Mogg had his father's face cast, wanting to preserve a three-dimensional portrait of the man for future generations; he liked the perman-ence of it, he liked having something solid and tangible. Mostly it's the faces of men, commissioned by their widows. But then there are the others, the people Nick won't name, the people who aren't famous, and may not be rich, despite the £2,500 price tag. Yesterday, he cast the cold feet of a five-week-old premature baby. Two weeks ago, the face of a fourteen-year-old cancer victim. Last year, a healthy twenty-six-year-old man who stepped backwards on a pavement and tripped.

'There's something about taking a mask of someone, whether you do believe the mystery of death passes off into it or not,' he says, back by the open window. 'The fact that it's still a unique face, and it's as unique as a person's fingerprints, and it's the last chance you're gonna get. I think, for a lot of people, it's just the case of knowing that they've managed to save a part of them that isn't going to become worm food or ashes. They suddenly realise that the person's gone and they want a part of them to stay. Whether there's any rational thinking to it at the actual time, or whether it's a last-chance-saloon thing, I don't know. Personally, I think they're great things, death masks. I think it's amazing that there's the person, dead, and you can just click your fingers, more or less, and they turn to stone. And you can keep that. Instead of it rotting on you.'

§

Nick tells me that when you die, you look amazing. All tension is released from your face, lines disappear, years of worry and pain vanish in moments. You look serene. Your face takes on an even colour. 'Ideally, I would get to them while they were still warm,' he says, small clouds escaping as he speaks. 'Weeks down the line, when I get the call, it's not really the same thing. They look a bit ... concertinaed.'

The Victorians believed that the sooner the death mask was taken, the more of a person you could capture; they would some-times call for the death mask maker before the doctor came to sign the death certificate. But Nick arrives when time and biology have shrunken skin and cartilage. When lips have shrivelled, the domes of the eyes have sunk, and the nose has started to twist. Perhaps there's an autopsy incision, maybe the skin has wrinkled like a prune as if the person spent too long in the pool. Maybe a drawn-out court case has left icicles to form on a body in a freezer. But he doesn't think there is any merit in handing someone a sculpture of their father as he looked after five weeks in a funeral home re-frigerator – it is not him as he was in life, just a consequence of the slow admin of death. So he nips, tucks, smooths. He massages the skin of the dead face back into place and then later, through sculpting and what he calls an obsessive attention to detail, he un-does the effects of gravity that cause cheeks to sink towards the ears, jowls to bunch under the jaw. 'Essentially, I try to get it to look as if I did it just after they died,' he says. 'I try to make it look as if I haven't done anything.'

Some people ask for the eyes to be opened, others can't make up their mind, but mostly they look like they're sleeping. Old death masks, like the Duke of Wellington's, let nature stand as it is. Lacking teeth, it looks like his lips are being pulled down his throat by an invisible hand. But he died in 1852, when real death was what was expected – not the image the modern-day em-balmer, or Nick, would perfect.

'The first thing you do is get their hair right,' he says, verbally walking me through a process that is now so automatic that he keeps having to stop and fill in bits he forgot to mention. Next, he covers their face in Nivea lotion, and positions the person so that the liquid rubber alginate isn't going to run down their neck, into their clothes. If he's lucky, they will be on a tray in the mor-tuary, wearing a paper hospital gown that will be changed anyway. But more often than not, they are already dressed in their burial

clothes and lying in their coffin, so Nick spends an hour meticulously placing black bin liners to protect the fabric, tucking them
like Kleenex into a newsreader's collar. The blue alginate, the same
used by dentists to take an impression of teeth, is poured over the
face and takes about two and a half minutes to set to the consistency of 'a sort of hard blancmange' – soft, flexible, it will collapse
or tear without something to reinforce it, so Nick forms a hard
casing around it with plaster bandages, as if setting a broken arm.
Twenty minutes later, he pulls the whole thing off. 'Nine times out
of ten, you actually lift the head up with it and have to shake the
head out,' he says. One time, a man's face came off attached to the
alginate: his features had been expensively reconstructed in wax
for the family's upcoming viewing, and now it was too late to get
the wax artist back to fix it. The panicked funeral director asked
Nick if he had any experience with reconstructive wax – he didn't,
but as a sculptor he had experience of wax in general, so he gave it
a go, recreating the nose, lips and eyes right there in the mortuary.
'I was shaking,' he says. 'I got away with it, but it was nowhere near
as good.'

With the cast in his wheelie bag, he cleans up the work area,
washes his bowls and picks any remaining bits of alginate from the
deceased's hair. Some funeral homes have told him it's not necessary, that the viewings had already happened so nobody would ever
know if he didn't stay and comb the hair until the dead looked like
they did before he arrived. But like Terry switching back the faces
in the Mayo, Nick would know. So he stays, he fixes it, and then he
rushes home to fill the mould before the rubber starts to shrink.

If there is minimal reconstruction work, he will fill it with
plaster and chisel any changes after it hardens. If the face needs
more attention, he will fill the mould with wax, which is mal-
leable – if all he needs to do is straighten a dehydrated, twisted
nose, he can gently push it straight before the wax has cooled.
The plaster or wax face is then moulded again in painted layers of
silicon rubber before that mould is, finally, filled with polyurethane
resin mixed with a metal powder. The heavy metal sinks through
the resin to the surface of the cast, creating an outer layer the

thickness of three cigarette papers. Transfer after transfer, several prints away from the original flesh face: a permanent, incorrupt-ible one in bronze.

You can see Nick's process for making a death mask in a grainy three-minute video on YouTube. It's not as neat as the situation laid out above, but the circumstances weren't as neat either. In 2007, he travelled to Texas for the execution, by lethal injection, of thirty-two-year-old John Joe Amador, convicted thirteen years previously for the murder of a taxi driver. 'I was convinced that the guy was innocent,' said Nick, who had been introduced to Amador's story by a mutual friend. 'I was outraged that he had been on death row for twelve years and had lost every appeal, even though the evidence was laughable.' He suggested to the friend that he go with her to the execution, and make a death mask as a way of raising public awareness about the horror and injustice of the death penalty. He wanted to cast Amador's arm too, and later add three hypodermic needles jutting from the vein.

After the execution, Nick, along with Amador's family, took his body from the prison morgue (who would not allow a cast to be taken on the premises – 'They said, "Nope, you can't do that, are you crazy?!"'), put him in the flattened back seat of a rental car and drove him to a cabin in the woods – a pit stop on the way to another funeral home they claimed they had waiting in order to gain release of the body, but at that point didn't. 'Basically, we'd kidnapped this body to take it to a little hut like in Friday the 13th, and we were all shitting ourselves, paranoid, thinking we're gonna get nicked by the FBI,' he says. 'It took us about ten hours to drive there, in a two-car convoy. One of the cars got picked up by the Old Bill at one point. Luckily, it was the one without the body in it. That would've been quite tricky to explain.'

On the drive, they unzipped the body bag so his wife could hold his hand. It was the first time he had been touched by friends or family in twelve years of incarceration. He was still warm.

It was hot in Texas, and hotter still in the cabin. Nick worried that his limited amount of alginate would set too quickly – luke-warm water can make it set in the bowl while you're mixing it – so he used ice-cold water and worked fast, casting his face and arm at the same time, trying to outrun the effects of the ambient temperature. When he pulled the mould off half an hour later, the chill of the alginate had given the dead man goosebumps.

Nick walks out of the sitting room and comes back with John Joe Amador's terracotta-coloured face on the back of a sculpture of an armadillo, the emblem of the state that killed him. 'The fact he was warm made me feel he was more real, I think,' he says, handing me the face before sinking into the sofa. 'When they've been dead for two weeks I don't feel that the person is there anymore. When they're warm it's almost as if – if there is such a thing – their spirit is lingering.' I run my fingers over Amador's chin and they are unmistakable: goosebumps on a dead man, like an amputated lizard's tail still writhing in the grass. Like a beheaded turtle, snapping.

'I spoke to him just before they killed him,' Nick says. 'He was over the moon, actually. He said, "Wow, you're the guy who's going to do my death mask. That's an honour they usually only reserve for people like kings. I used to think I was trash. Now I know I'm someone."'

§

When the police eventually caught up with his father – bursting through the front door when Nick was only six – Bruce went to one prison for twenty-five years and Nick to another: boarding school. During this otherwise miserable time, he remembers a school trip to Warwick Castle, standing in a room full of portraits of Oliver Cromwell. He was puzzled by how different they all were and, with art as his favourite subject, he wondered if artists were just worse back then, or if, despite famously asking to be painted warts and all, they were pandering to Cromwell's vanity. With these questions in his mind, he turned to leave and saw, there on the wall, Cromwell's death mask. Nick was able to judge for himself what was true.

Decades later, he was at his parents' house, paging through a book on sculpture. It was 1995. While his father watched Ronnie Kray's funeral on the television, Nick read a section on mould-making, a detailed tutorial on how to take a cast of a person's face. The news kept flickering on the screen in the background, the elaborate goodbye to a criminal icon that Nick knew from childhood prison visits as just another guy in a cell beside his father. 'I was completely taken aback that his funeral was attended by so many people,' he says. 'I thought it was interesting how the media can turn people into icons even if they're criminals.' His own father's robbery was originally called the Cheddington Mail Van Raid until the press sensationalised it, dubbing it the Great Train Robbery. They made heroes out of thieves. 'This kind of resonated in my mind. So I thought, *Why don't I do an exhibition on the paradox of how villains are basically slagged off in the media on one hand, and are on the celebrity circuit the next?*' Nick, who isn't ashamed of what his father did but isn't exactly proud of it, asked his father to write him a list of the ten most infamous living criminals. He was going to cast their faces and call the exhibition *Cons to Icons*.

Despite their historical link to royalty, there is also a long history of casting death masks of criminals for a very different reason. In the nineteenth century, casting the full heads of criminals was once an integral part in the study of phrenology – the long-debunked science of figuring out a person's psychology, and by extension their biological inclination towards crime and violence, through the bumps on their skull. In Scotland Yard's Black Museum (a collection not open to the public, housing criminal memorabilia originally intended to help in the training of police) there are death masks of those executed outside Newgate prison – Daniel Good, who murdered his wife, and Robert Marley, who bludgeoned to death the owner of a jewellery store, among others. Just down the hall from Jeremy Bentham's clothed skeleton at UCL are thirty-seven masks they don't know what to do with, remnants of a long-dead phrenologist's collection. Some bear the axe wounds of the imprecise executioner's first attempts. Others, the imprint of the hangman's noose.

But Nick wasn't casting dead criminals – these men were still alive. He used his father as a guinea pig, accidentally leaving him with acid burns from a lemon he held in his mouth so that Nick could depict him swallowing a golden train in the finished piece ('My dad had a romantic idea of himself as Captain Ahab choking on Moby Dick'). Next, he flew to Brazil to cast Ronnie Biggs. Then, he nearly killed 'Mad' Frankie Fraser, a violent gangland criminal whose trademark torture method was to nail victims to the floor and extract their teeth with gold-plated pliers, a habit which earned him the moniker 'The Dentist'. Fraser couldn't breathe through the straws, as his nose had been broken so many times it barely worked as a nose. 'When I noticed his knuckles had gone white and he was shaking, I asked him if he was all right. He obviously didn't hear me through all the plaster I'd put over his head, so in a panic I pulled everything off and there he was, gasping. He was holding his breath, rather than put up a signal and give in! I thought that was the measure of the man.' In the finished sculpture, Nick has Mad Frankie – an inmate officially certified insane no less than three times, although he claimed he faked it for more lenient punishment – in a straitjacket.

At the top of his father's list was George 'Taters' Chatham, his father's mentor, and a man once described by the *Guardian* as 'the Thief of the Century'. But he was having trouble tracking him down. When he finally found him, he was dead – but only very recently so. Nick got in touch with Chatham's sister and asked if he could do a cast of him anyway. It would be just like a life mask, only they would have no need for the straws. A broken nose, if he had one, wouldn't matter.

Chatham's sister thought it was an odd request, but told Nick she was going to view him at the funeral home that afternoon and would let him know how she felt. Later that evening, he got a call. She said he was smiling, so he'd obviously made his peace with God – she was happy for him to take the cast.

'The next day I went to the morgue for the first time. It was the first time I'd met him too, which was quite strange. And I did what was my first death mask. He was, indeed, smiling,' says Nick. 'I didn't tell her that was only because of the weight of the jowls.'

§

After boarding school, Nick joined the Navy. It was partly because his father had always wanted to but was rejected after a failed eye test, and also because a job on the move didn't sound too far from the life he already knew, having spent his formative years as a fugitive. He served four years on HMS *Hermes* (named after the Greek god of, among other things, thieves) in the Falklands, as an electronic weapons engineer and a diver, before being drafted to a landlocked post. Not being able to dive meant he wasn't able to earn his diver's pay, which required him to spend a certain number of hours underwater – like pilots and flight. So he joined the Thames Wapping Police Underwater Unit to make up the time. Despite the realities of war – of seeing people in pieces, bleeding – Nick says the Falklands had nothing on what the police divers were regularly confronted with, every day, in their own city.

'They were a bunch of lunatics,' says Nick. 'They were all drunk from 9 a.m. onwards, and I soon learned why. They see some pretty fucking horrible things. Sometimes it's a gun in the river, or a car in the river, but mostly it's a body. The very first time I went with them, they stuck me in a lake to identify whether a driver was still in the car, and to put a chain around the bumper. As much as I tried not to look through the window of the car, I did. He didn't look too good.'

I ask if being around the dead, if seeing the dead as they truly are, makes him think differently about dying. Or if it gets to him, this slow parade of dead faces on the kitchen bench.

'There's only so much I can carry around in my head,' he says, the ceiling now overcast. 'I had a pretty brutal childhood, particularly going through boarding school. I'm very good at compartmentalising things and shutting them off, but that's probably the nature of my life. Everyone can do it, but maybe I've just been in situations where I've had to learn how to do it more, and I've become very good at it. I can hold things at bay. I can shut doors in my head if I have to. Although, that generally means that I have to do it by focusing on something else. I've always got so much going on, so that's not a problem for me – or maybe that is a problem. One of my kids said to me once that I'm running away from reality by having so much to do that I don't really have any time to consider reality.'

'If you did have time to think, would it be bad?' I remember the Shirley Jackson line at the beginning of *The Haunting of Hill House*, that 'no live organism can continue for long to exist sanely under conditions of absolute reality'. I wonder how much reality, and for how long, it would take to crush someone.

'I don't think it would be beneficial. It would get you down if you think about death all the time. Particularly if it was a suicide – why did they do it? There's too much living to do to dwell too much on the dead. There's nothing good about being wrapped up in death all the time. It can make you melancholic.'

I ask, if he does not want to dwell on the dead, why he has chosen an art that means he comes face to face with one of the realities he is supposedly running from by being so busy. Why he works for days, months, on something so quiet, when the rest of his life is lived so loudly.

'A lot of what I do is all very trivial and quite selfish,' he says. 'Even though it broke my heart doing the little girl's feet yesterday, it made me feel that at least my life isn't just one rollercoaster of me having fun all the time.' He reminds me now of Poppy, seeking something more nourishing than selling paintings in an auction house. 'I'm doing something that's very valid,' he says. 'Most of the art I do, it's all egotistical; being in the band, it's all ego. I think what I'm doing is very, very worthwhile. I wouldn't do it otherwise. It's kind of a calling. There isn't anyone else doing it, and I think if there was I'd more likely say, "It doesn't have to be me." Everything else I do is because I want to do it. It's good to have something that I don't particularly want to do, but I feel that I should.'

Nick would, given the choice, rather cast the living, despite believing there is no spiritual power in a life mask. He would rather the nips and tucks he does to make a person look less dead or sunken were not required. But people, if they think about it at all, only think about it after the fact. They want to preserve the essence of a life only when that life has gone, so there is always an element of sadness in a death mask; they exist only because of a loss. Nick looks up at the life mask of his father, once one of the most wanted criminals in the world, and says he thinks, sometimes, about swapping it for the death mask that sits on his headstone in Highgate Cemetery, and has a tendency to look sad in the shade. Something in the recess of the eyes, something in the gravity that pulls the features downward. His father's death was five years ago and he still finds it painful to talk about. He avoids it for most of the time I am with him, looking away to roll cigarettes, asking if I have other questions. But just before I leave, he tells me he wishes now that he hadn't propped him up in his chair – it's not how he usually works, and he can't remember now why he did it that way; finding his father dead and the months that followed were a blur. He struggles still to recall them, locked as they are somewhere behind a door in his mind. But the life mask would slot just as neatly into the space where the death mask sits, there between the hand-carved quote on the left –*THIS IS IT!* – the words his father spoke into the walkie-talkie as he lifted his ear off the railway track that night in 1963, and those on the right – *C'EST LA VIE!* – as he was arrested.

The next time I visited Highgate Cemetery – on a wintery day where the hellebores pitched sideways in a gale so strong it made the trees above me creak – I noticed a little seat had been tucked in front of the headstone. Just a small piece of wood balanced on stones. It was invisible from the main path, obscured by the mound of another grave. I sat down, and I was eye-level with Nick's father, a face that looks strikingly like Nick's own. The rain trickled down his bronze skin, its path rerouted by the delicate wrinkles formed over a lifetime.

Limbo

The Kenyon offices are in a forgettable brick building out on a bleak industrial plane on the fringes of London where everything is either roundabout or car park. There is nothing here but huge shops that sell stuff to fix your car, your house, your garden – everything that makes your life look good from the outside. Halfords Autocentre, Wickes, Homebase. A visibly derelict but apparently still functioning bowling alley called Hollywood Bowl rises above a shabby Pizza Hut. Everything is mostly tarmac bar the self-conscious attempts at beautifying the concrete with landscaping: a pond with a short bridge over it and a sign on a tree stump telling you how beautiful all of this is. Someone in a hi-vis yellow vest waves to me from the other end of another car park: 'Yes, this is the place,' the wave says – the place in question being chosen for its proximity to Heathrow Airport and nothing else. There is no time to waste in a mass fatality, wherever in the world it might be.

I'd never heard of Kenyon – a company whose logo subtitle says 'International Emergency Services', which is sort of vague about what it is, exactly, that they do – but Iwan, the company's operations manager, tells me there's a good reason for my ignorance: I'm not supposed to have heard of Kenyon. 'We're a white-label company. When you phone up for information after a disaster, we're working on behalf of a client. We take their name,' he says, as he places a plate of Party Rings and a cup of tea on the glass coffee table in the reception area. I found them when I was looking around for a detective to interview – a lot of ex-police end up here. But it's not like Kenyon and what they do are a secret.

Their website is full of stories by people who work there, talking about things they've done, places they've been deployed. He leaves me with a pile of magazines: the *Funeral Service Times*, the *Aeronautical Journal*, *Insight: The Voice of Independent Funeral Directors* and *Airliner World*. I'm at the intersection of a Venn diagram.

When a disaster happens, when your plane crashes or your building burns or your train T-bones a bus, Kenyon will assume your company's name and work in tandem with the local authorities to deal with the aftermath. They will respond to the media for you, making sure your message is clear and consistent so that your staff can concentrate on the internal implosion that is likely occurring. They will fix your website so that if, for example, the co-pilot deliberately ploughed your Germanwings plane into the Alps, killing all 144 passengers plus the six crew members, there are no glossy photographs of the Alps on your page promoting travel on your low-cost airline while emergency workers are picking through the wreckage on the mountain.

Kenyon will set up a crisis line that people can phone to register the missing and inquire about developments. They will provide family liaison officers to translate the horror into something true but manageable, one familiar voice instead of a company that speaks to them en masse through a megaphone. They will set up the 'dark side' of your website, where families can log in and be given information in real time, and a family assistance centre where they can sit and wait and be, where they can pray on the book of their chosen religion, have access to mental-health practitioners, and hear announcements made in every language that needs to be heard.

Kenyon make travel arrangements for families affected and move people from the farthest reaches of the earth to the place where their loved one died, whether that requires a plane, a train, or a horse and cart to fetch them from the deepest forest in Brazil. They secure accommodation, quietly ensuring the hotel doesn't also have a wedding with 400 guests at the same time as the media briefing on a plane crash, and organise staggered mealtimes so that grieving families are not eating at the same time as holiday guests. They will organise the memorials: over a hundred years of experience in managing disasters (their first was in 1906, when a boat train jumped its tracks and crashed in Salisbury, England) means Kenyon knows that every disaster is different, and how each culture deals with death and dead bodies is different; they know that giving roses to Japanese families to place on their dead is improper – white chrysanthemums are preferred. Every practical problem that comes up has already been considered and dealt with, including the likelihood of media faking ID cards to sneak into the family assistance centre for tabloid scoops: in 2010, when a runway crash at a Libyan airport resulted in 103 dead, a reporter was arrested for doing just this. If the disaster is a fire, they will have already requested that the catering crew steer clear of barbecued meat.

They've thought of everything you haven't, and won't, because you're in the midst of a catastrophe and this probably hasn't happened to you, or your company, before.

I'm here for Kenyon's open day, where they are selling – this is, after all, a commercial enterprise – a step-by-step solution to a problem that hasn't arrived yet. There are dozens of people here today representing all kinds of companies that see mass fatality as a very real possibility in their futures: airlines, local councils, service industries, rail companies, bus companies, fire services, shipping companies, oil and gas companies. Over the course of seven hours, Kenyon is going to explain why these businesses need to sign up with them now, before the bad thing happens. They're going to explain why having a plan in place is essential, not only to the families and to staff, but to the company name. Malaysian Airlines will crop up repeatedly as a cautionary tale, an airline that will likely never recover from their two crashes in 2014 that left a death toll of 537. As we sit on fold-out chairs, clutching paper bags with Kenyon-branded stationery, surrounded by model aeroplanes balanced on windowsills, we are told that people on the whole can accept a disaster. They can grieve their lost loved ones and can handle grim truth better than you think. But they cannot and will not accept an inadequate response from a company that had no plan for the living or the dead.

§

Mark Oliver, or 'Mo' as everyone calls him, is fifty-three. If the police were to describe him they would say he was average height, average build, glasses, with grey hair short and neat enough to be military. He wears a suit to work except when he's deployed to a disaster: there he'll be wearing something from his go-bag that he keeps ready and waiting in the sprawling warehouse out the back of the Kenyon office. He takes me through a door with a laminated piece of white A4 that says in all red-and-black caps: *STOP! CHECK! ARE YOU DIRTY???* to a line of tall, grey school lockers near shelves bearing folded embalming tables stacked ten deep above portable embalming kits. He opens a locker and perfunctorily shows off large evidence bags repurposed to allow ease of packing, each holding clothes for climates hot, cold, wet, dry. Everything is neatly folded, enough in each bag for a week or so, enough time to get a plan in place to have more clothes sent to wherever he needs to be. He opens another locker and points. 'There,' he says, laughing, 'now you've seen my boss's underpants.'

Mo joined Kenyon in 2014 and became VP of operations in 2018. He's responsible for their field operations, training and consultancy, as well as managing their vast list of team members. Among the 2,000 people on the Kenyon payroll are people who previously worked in aviation, psychologists specialising in grief and PTSD, firefighters, forensic scientists, radiographers, former Naval officers, police officers, detective constables and a former commander of New Scotland Yard. There are crisis-management specialists with experience in crises both air travel- and banking-related, embalmers and funeral directors, retired pilots, bomb disposal specialists and an advisor to the Mayor of London. If you were putting together an apocalypse crew, you could do worse than this. Add a surgeon and you'd probably survive with the cockroaches and the deep sea fish.

Prior to all of this, Mo spent thirty years in the police service across the UK. As a senior investigating officer he worked
on homicides, organised crime, anti-corruption and counter-
terrorism. Despite his serious role, Mo is a joker. Not quite in the
same flippant way that Baltimore cops in David Simon's *Homicide*
pasted angel wings to the backs of dead drug dealer mugshots and
hung them from their Christmas tree, but that humour you find in
the bleakest of places is present and accounted for in Mo. It needs
to be – humour sustains, and here at Kenyon it carries a consid-
erable load: we're in the same warehouse as thousands of items
that belonged to the tenants of Grenfell Tower, the burned-out
apartment block that loomed black and skeletal over west London
until the authorities covered it up with a giant tarpaulin and hoped
we'd look away. It doesn't matter how far away from the burning
of Grenfell Tower we get, 14 June 2017 still feels like a fresh
wound. Seventy-two people died, seventy were injured, and 223
people escaped from this fire that highlighted the political and social failings of the system, high and low. As the inquest rolled on,
Kenyon was still picking through the personal belongings of those
in the building and trying to locate the families at their new, temporary addresses in order to return them. From almost all of the
129 flats, something was found. Some 750,000 individual items
were boxed up and brought back from North Kensington to be
processed here, then cleaned and returned. It was still happening
two years later, in 2019, when I visited Kenyon.

Earlier, I watched Mo explain the power and significance of
personal effects to people who would have to explain that same
power to the people who control the money, who have the au-
thority to say whether or not it is worth shelling out for their
recovery. Personal effects are not just *stuff*; he tells us that within
an item that somebody had with them at the time they met their
end there is untold emotional weight, and it is not for us to judge
how heavy. Traditionally, local authorities aren't too bothered with
personal effects; police might stick them in a cupboard and forget
about them, or pass them to someone else who might forget about
them too (I once worked with an investigative journalist who had

a murder victim's clothes in a plastic bag in his desk drawer that he intended to return, but it wasn't a priority). But death is transformative, not just to the person and the family; it changes the objects in a house. These objects become, as Maggie Nelson wrote in The Red Parts – a book about the murder of her aunt and the subsequent trial – talismans.

Now Mo is walking me through the aisles of things found inside Grenfell, boxes stacked high above us. 'It was crammed before,' he says, of a warehouse I would still classify as crammed. There may be a lot less here than there used to be, but it still takes over most of the place. Thousands of cardboard boxes line the shelves, and things that are too large to fit in a box are stacked in their categories by the wall: pushbikes ranging from a child's BMX to an adult-size racer, prams, bouncy things you put babies in while the twirling mobile dazzles them into silence. Suitcases. High chairs, singed and not. To the front of the warehouse is the processing department: Kenyon will ask, if an item is being returned, whether the family want it cleaned, be it a toy car, pyjama bottoms or a coin. 'If you'd been here earlier you would have seen washing lines strung up across the aisles,' he says, grinning and spreading his arms out like a scarecrow – they'd done a panic-tidy before the open day. There are bottles of cleaning products on the shelves, hair dryers, multiple irons. Just off this area of the warehouse is the photography room, where gridded A4 pages show examples of how to photograph different items, from pens to bras, to sweaters with an arm folded, the other outstretched.

Back in the reception area I had flipped through a binder of 'unassociated personal effects' – photographs, taken here, of items from other disasters that never did find their owners but are still filed away somewhere with an ID number, waiting. Standing there, among open-day attendees eating triangular sandwiches off paper plates and fussing with a tea urn, I found it haunting. The personal item next to the systematic code, the thickness of the binder, thousands of meaningless things filled with meaning for someone unknown. Tortoiseshell reading glasses with a frame warped by fire or explosion or both, keys to houses and Alfa Romeos, prayer cards. A bloated Ian Rankin novel pulled from the sea.

When the family has been identified and contacted and they are absolutely sure they don't want the item back, whatever it may be needs to be rendered unidentifiable before it is thrown away. Mo takes me to the back of the warehouse, to a different department, where six people in white jumpsuits and protective visors smash nineties VHS tapes with hammers, the careful Sharpie lettering along the stickers visible in a gloved hand before it is obliterated. He's shouting over the noises of hammers hitting plastic, of pieces flying and landing nearby, some joke about paid stress relief, but I can't quite hear him. I see episodes of *Friends* taped over episodes of *Taggart*. I see tapes that look exactly like tapes I have at home that hold irreplaceable footage of childhood. In among the shards, a Britney Spears CD.

Three months after the flames were extinguished, Kenyon workers, still combing through the charred remains, found a fish tank in the blackened tower. Somehow, despite the lack of food, electricity to oxygenate their water, and the twenty-three dead fish floating belly up above them, seven fish still lived. The family from the flat were contacted but were unable to house them in their current situation, so with their blessing, one of the Kenyon staff adopted the fish. They even managed to breed, resulting in the most unlikely thing to rise from the ashes of a burned building: a baby fish.

They called it Phoenix.

§

It was never the plan to end up here: Mo was retired from the police force when he was offered the role. But two decades ago, he took part in an operation that would set the current course.

It was 2000, the year after the controversial eleven-week bombing campaign by NATO to end the Kosovo War, and international help was arriving to investigate the atrocities. Intelligence reports located mass graves, and forensic teams carried out exhumations and post-mortems, and tried to identify the dead to reunite them with their families. They needed someone urgently to fill in for five weeks. Mo was, at that point, running homicide investigations, specifically unsolved murders. He was used to going to post-mortems, he was used to being organised, and he could set up the computer systems they needed for an undertaking this huge – the skills that made him a good police officer made him an ideal candidate for the job. 'I flew over there, got given the keys to a Land Rover, and the next day they sent me a team of thirty people to brief.' His eyes bug out as he's telling me now: mass graves in Kosovo were a world away from Hendon, north London. 'Crikey,' he says.

Four years later, when the tsunami hit Sri Lanka on Boxing Day, the Metropolitan Police were sending people over to help identify the thousands of dead. Mo had successfully identified people in Kosovo – from the fully skeletonised, to the hardly touched – so they sent him, putting him in charge of the process across all nationalities. Mo was there for six months, getting very little sleep. All the while, he was meeting other disaster response people, working with the same guys who would eventually, years later, pull him out of his brief police retirement and give him a permanent role here at Kenyon.

It's a couple of weeks after the open day and everything here is quieter now. We're sitting in his office and Mo is talking me through some of the other cases he's worked on: the Germanwings crash into the Alps in 2015, the mass shooting in Tunisia that left thirty-eight dead in 2015, the 2016 Egyptair Flight 804 that plummeted into the Mediterranean Sea killing everyone on board, and the Emirates plane that crashed at Dubai airport in 2016 but killed just one person on the ground. He says the most obvious failing in every airline's disaster response plan, if they have one, is they all expect the crash to happen at their own airport. No one accounts for the infrastructure or wealth, or lack of each, of another country.

There are framed photos of his time in the police, and knick-knacks on the shelves beside mass fatality manuals. I point at one, a beaten-up padlock with a scuffed handwritten label hanging on a small varnished wooden stand, and ask about it. 'That's the padlock that we took off on the last day in Sri Lanka,' he says, as he brings it down off the shelf and places it between us on the table. It came from one of the forty-foot refrigerated shipping containers – like the kind you see on the back of a lorry – that held the unidentified bodies recovered after the tsunami in 2004. When the last body was identified, when the containers, after six harrowing months, were empty, the coroner of Sri Lanka gifted him the final padlock. 'It was a pretty significant time for us all,' he says, 'to realise that we'd got through the task and we'd laid those people to rest.'

A total of 227,898 people died in the tsunami as the colossal waves rolled over coastlines in Indonesia, Thailand, India, Sri Lanka and South Africa. Over thirty thousand died in Sri Lanka alone. The local authorities moved quickly to bury the bodies – fearing that leaving them where they lay, in the tropical heat, would be a health hazard to the living. They put them in mass graves, many beside hospitals, with a view to them being exhumed by international authorities in search of their own. 'The authorities in Sri Lanka didn't want to go through a mass identification for their nationals,' explains Mo. 'Many were Buddhists, Hindus – they were happy that those people had been buried in mass graves. But by the same token, the authorities and the government there knew that the foreigners wouldn't understand that culture. They wouldn't want to be left in those graves. So they tried to preserve where the obvious foreigners were buried, and said they would work with us to identify them.'

Rotating teams of UK police and forensic officers investigated where the mass graves containing foreigners might be and exhumed them. About 300 bodies filled the seven refrigerated containers, all unidentified, awaiting post-mortems. Ante-mortem information – meaning pre-death – was collected across the nationalities to match up to the bodies in the containers: dental, DNA, fingerprints. But collecting ante-mortem information for hundreds of missing foreigners is no small feat: at the Kenyon open day, Mo had shown us how it was done. He had told us that you don't know what state the body will be in if and when you find it, so you need every piece of information you can get, about every piece of that body. It's great if somebody has a tattoo on their arm, but what if you don't find their arm? Similarly, you might think a tattoo is unique, and then discover – as with a Wile E. Coyote tattoo in a past case – that it's the mascot of a Marine Transport Squadron and hundreds of men have it. The co-mingling of personal effects in an explosion or crash means a wallet with an ID card found on a body might not be that body's wallet. You have to question everything. As an exercise, Mo had made us team up with the person beside us and role play the collection of ante-mortem information. He told us to record any medical implants – pacemakers, breasts – citing their unique and traceable serial numbers as invaluable: he recently identified someone on the basis of a prosthetic patella. That is to say, the most identifiable part of the man was his kneecap. In the role play, I pretended to be my mother providing information on me, and the quiet fire warden beside me assumed the role of Kenyon staff. I counted the two screws in each leg from knee surgeries, a faded birthmark on my left thigh, the scar on my wrist from when I smashed a window in a teenage rage, and the white line on my shoulder from when I crashed my pink tricycle into a wheelie bin. It's here, answering questions that might help in my body's identification, that I realise I don't tell my family anything: they don't know who my GP is, my dentist, they don't know if or when I've had blood samples taken or needed medical intervention, they don't know if I've submitted my DNA to some genetic ancestry test like 23andMe, or whether I've ever needed a fingerprint to enter a building I work in. I pictured my parents offering the family liaison officer patchy bits of information like fluff from their pockets. I pictured mortuary staff sorting through the pieces, trying to find those childhood scars. It seemed, to me, to be an expensive undertaking, in both money and time.

'Was it purely out of religious reasons that the local authorities were content to leave their own unidentified?' I ask Mo now in his office. 'Or was it because the victims were poor?'

'There's definitely a political aspect,' he says. 'Far fewer people died in Thailand, yet there was a huge international effort in Thailand. Why? Because they decided to try and identify *everyone*, and that took eighteen months to two years to do. How much of that was because so many of the people there were rich tourists?' He gives a small shrug, as if to say it always comes down to money, and the money isn't always up to him. 'That meant there was more international focus on them. Politics is completely involved in the funding and the approach to a disaster.'

Another case where the poverty of the locals came into play was the Philippines. Typhoon Haiyan, one of the most powerful tropical cyclones ever recorded, made landfall in November 2013, when it threw cars like stones, flattened buildings and washed whole towns away. It killed at least 6,300 people in the Philippines alone. A city administrator estimated that 90 per cent of the city of Tacloban had been obliterated. This was where Mo and his team headed in the immediate wake of the storm: a ruined city so devastated that two years later Pope Francis would visit and lead mass for 30,000 people in front of the airport as a hope-raising exercise.

I tell Mo that I remember reading in the *New York Times* that bodies were left out for weeks, and he looks away like he still doesn't believe what he saw. 'Hayley, I've got pictures,' he says. He steps behind his desk and, after some searching and cursing – 'Jesus, how many bloody presentations have I done in my time?' – brings up a PowerPoint display on his computer. Here are the operation headquarters: the disused building with one toilet, with the tents and flimsy gazebos that served as their temporary mortuary, put up by local authorities using whatever they could find. There were no official temporary mortuary supplies in the area, and no refrigeration. 'I ♥ TACLOBAN' is printed on one of the gazebos. Beside it, a marshy field, dense with mosquitoes, where body bags were lined up in their thousands, bursting in the heat. The rate of decomposition in a place as hot as Tacloban was high – the average temperature at the time was 27 degrees Celsius, with humidity at 84 per cent – and the gases were causing the plastic to tear, spilling contents into puddles in the field. I ask Mo what the smell was like and he pauses, like he's never stopped to consider it. 'I don't think I've got a very good sense of smell, actually,' he says, looking up from his screen. 'It probably helps in my job. Although, in Sri Lanka, there was the sweet smell of death for a whole fourteen-hour car journey.'

Further on, more photographs: here's Mo personally fishing three bodies out of a lagoon in the Philippines. The typhoon didn't leave the bodies here: it was a local policeman trying to help. The bodies had been out in the open, decomposing – he was trying to save the survivors from the smell, the sight, the horror. So he disposed of them in the nearest water source, succeeding only in poisoning it for everyone nearby. They're bloated, pale, face down in the water. Using two planks of wood, one at the pelvis, the other under the arms, a limp body is lifted out and brought to the shore by kayak. The skin along the back is smooth and puffy, but the front of the body is skeletal, the face nibbled off by creatures. 'We've recovered air-disaster victims with shark bites taken out of them,' said Mo, clicking through the slides – nature just gets on with it. Here are the bodies laid out on a tarpaulin. Here's Mo lifting the leg of a victim, pointing at the blue rope that the policeman thought would tie the body to the bottom of the lagoon and make it disappear.

He's clicking through the photographs faster now, trying to show me what he means when he said he looked across the field of body bags and thought to himself, *I don't think I'll solve this one.* These photos were taken a week after the storm took those lives, and already the bags are full of brown soup, creamy ribcages jutting above the slop, maggots visible in the mix. Skulls, stripped of their defining flesh features, lank hair pasted over cheek and eye. More bloated corpses in their swimming costumes, now so far from the beach. Adults, children. I've been listening to Mo talk about his job for hours, but in looking at these photos, only now can I begin to fathom how difficult identification is. These are not drowned people pulled from a lake: this is decaying meat and bone; there are no faces, let alone tattoos. On the positive side, at least this person is all here: they are not in forty-seven pieces picked from the rubble of a plane crash. This is not, in theory, a hopeless situation – bodies like this can still be matched by DNA or dental records. But Typhoon Haiyan took not only their lives but their houses, and with them any possible chance of collecting ante-mortem information that could have been matched up with the dead: any strands of hair, any toothbrushes that could be mined for genetic code, any mirrors or door handles recording the unique whorls of their fingerprints. And the poorer the person, the less likely they are to visit a dentist. No one here beeped their way into a high-rise office building by pressing their thumb to a scanner.

Nevertheless, there was a mortuary team from the Philippines working through the thousands of dead at a rate of about fifteen people per day, collecting post-mortem information that would never, and likely could never, be matched up to information that might identify them. They were going through the motions without considering whether any of it would mean anything. Mo decided it was inhumane to leave these bodies rotting for as long as the local authorities did: there was no proper plan in place for identification, no international government interest, and therefore no money. It was needless horror in a situation that was already emotionally sensitive to the survivors.

'Full respect to those who were trying it, but I identified it as being an impossible task. I tried to get them to bury them in individual graves, maybe take a tooth or something,' he says – a tooth being the easiest thing to keep, a vague hope that maybe some identification might be possible rather than nothing at all. 'In the end, all the internationals went home for Christmas, and they brought in the JCBs, the big digging machines, and buried them. They realised they couldn't do any more.'

§

Months ago in south London we carefully laid Adam out in the spring-lit mortuary, delicately removing and folding his T-shirt for his family to collect. Thinking back to him now, sitting here with

Mo, I am struck by the huge gulf between what 'methodical' means in a quiet, expected death and 'methodical' in a mass-fatality situation – the consideration of the individual versus what is the best you can do with what you've got. It changes with every disaster, but there are some fundamentals that are immovable – all learned, as with most of these things, through what others did wrong.

In 1989, a boat sank on the Thames. It was the *Marchioness*, a small party boat that once helped rescue men in the 1940 Dunkirk evacuation. It collided with a huge dredger called the *Bowbelle* in the middle of the night, took thirty seconds to sink, left fifty-one dead (most of them under the age of thirty) and led to an official change in the way bodies were treated in the aftermath of a disaster, because the aftermath itself was a disaster too. According to Richard Shepherd, the forensic pathologist in charge of London and south-east England at the time, it was one of a series of disasters that revolutionised things: train collisions, shooting sprees, a lit match dropped through an escalator at King's Cross Station (every week I walk past a plaque in the station commemorating the people who died there). All of these and more led to the deaths of hundreds and exposed major systems failures. Corporate and state attitudes to training, risk and responsibility, health and safety – everything had to be overhauled.

Mo didn't work on the *Marchioness* case; he was a young police constable on a different patch when it happened. But pulling a binder off his bookshelf, *Public Inquiry into the Identification of Victims following Major Transport Accidents: Report of Lord Justice Clarke*, released eleven years after the *Marchioness* disaster, he explains how the sinking of that boat sent ripples through the following decades. At the root of it was the removal of the victims' hands.

'When homeless people – we used to call them vagrants in those days – fell into the Thames, and were fished out maybe two or three days later, they would be quite bloated and unrecognisable,' Mo explains. 'As anyone would be, in the water.' Death, however recent, changes how people look, which is why relying solely on visual identification is neither possible nor wise. According to the forensic pathologist Bernard Knight

CBE, who is quoted in the report, it's a common occurrence for close relatives to have doubts about, deny or mistakenly agree to the identity of a deceased person – even in freshly dead bodies. The effects of gravity on the features, the flattening of parts of the body that had contact with hard surfaces, swelling and pallor all work to distort the person as you might have known them. When the dynamic element of a person is gone – how they held their face, how they moved and made eye contact – sometimes what is left is unrecognisable.

Generally speaking, the kind of person who would be pulled out of the Thames tended to be someone who had been picked up by the police while alive – their fingerprints were already on the database, so they could, theoretically, be identified by prints alone in a short amount of time. But when a body has been in the water, it's not so easy a task: the skin becomes wrinkly like it does after a long bath, it turns white no matter what your ethnicity. Fingerprints become invisible. 'So what they'd do is they would remove the hands,' says Mo. 'They'd then take the hands to a drying cabinet in a fingerprint laboratory. After the hands had dried out, they could take the fingerprints.'

What happened in the *Marchioness* investigation was they applied small-time identification tactics on a massive scale, and to a group of people who were unlikely to have had their fingerprints on the database. The waterlogged skin was loosening and beginning to detach from the fingers, so it was becoming harder to get the prints they believed they needed. A laboratory in Southwark had more sophisticated fingerprinting equipment than the mortuary, but there were no facilities to handle the bodies. So, as with the individual cases of bodies in the Thames, they took only the hands.

The removal of the hands snowballed into larger problems: uninformed families seeing the bodies of their dead inexplicably handless, and mortuaries finding lost hands in the corners of freezers years after the rest of the body had been buried or cremated. 'They were carrying out processes to lead to the identification all in good faith, but it probably wasn't done in a coordinated way,' figures Mo, and his reasoning is backed up in Clarke's inquiry. Fifty-six pages of the Clarke report investigate every step that led to the decision to sever the hands. The other 200 or so are laying out guiding principles for the future: how bodies should be identified, who has the power to do what, and how the bereaved families are to be treated and what they are to be told.

'Now we'll have what's called an identification standard. Usually DNA, fingerprints, dental will be sufficient on their own as long as there are no exclusionary factors and no unexplainable discrepancies – I've had DNA back from people in the mortuary where I can see that it's a woman but a man's DNA has come back because of contamination. You have to consider all the pathology *in the round*.'

After the *Marchioness* disaster, some families were allowed to see their dead and others were refused access. Funeral directors and the police claimed that they were advised not to let the families see the bodies, even when the families were insistent that they wanted to. The pathologist, Shepherd, only learned about this later, and speculates that whoever made this decision probably did it with 'misplaced compassion' – the belief that seeing the body in its decomposed state would only upset the families more than they already were. 'However,' Shepherd wrote in his memoir *Unnatural Causes*, 'that person clearly did not know that *not* seeing them is even worse.'

I ask Mo about viewing the bodies. Given everything he's shown me, would he ever stop a family from seeing what he sees?

'In this country, there's a right for people to view bodies,' he says. 'It might be a body that is covered, and you just need to be there with them. Maybe part of the body or the face is shown. But because of the type of incidents that we deal with – which are high levels of fragmentations and perhaps the tiniest part of human remains – we will advise families, at an early stage, that the body is unlikely to be suitable for viewing. But we'll explain why, and that's not the same as denying them.'

In the explaining of why, family liaison officers have to be honest. After a plane crash, families are asked if they would like to be notified every time a new piece of a person is identified: would you like another call when they find the forty-seventh piece, or is the first one – the positive identification – enough? Some families might be offered a lock of hair to keep, but others might not. How can you offer a lock of hair if you do not find the head? Religious traditions might not be able to be carried out simply because there is not enough of the body there to do it. If you are not truthful about a situation, families cannot understand.

'In Egypt, after MS804, when I first got access to where the bodies were, sixty-six bodies were in three domestic five-drawer fridges. The largest body part was the size of an orange. And the most parts of human remains that were attributed to one individual were five. That did cause difficulties with the Muslim faith, when the family wanted to be present and wash the remains. *You are talking about a sample in a sample pot.* Nevertheless, the identification of someone and the presence of *some* of their body is very important.'

§

Back at the Kenyon open day, after a coffee break, Gail Dunham stepped up to the lectern to give a speech. She was a lady in her mid-seventies, with waves of neat grey hair and an array of brooches, both pretty and placard-y, decorating her lapels. She had been sitting alone all day, a few chairs away from various airline representatives, and stuck out as an anomaly in a room of suits. She is the executive director of the National Air Disaster Alliance/ Foundation, a group formed by the families of air crash survivors and victims to raise the standard of aviation safety, security and survivability, and to support victims' families. Kenyon were visibly thrilled to have her there, a straight-talking, polite woman who is both knowledgeable about the way the airlines work (she worked for American Airlines for twenty-seven years), and deeply familiar with how it feels to lose someone in a plane crash and be treated badly by the airline. In March 1991, United Airlines Flight 585, a Boeing 737-200, was approaching Colorado Springs to land when it rolled to the right, pitched nose-down until near vertical and hit the ground. Footage from the crash site, a local park south of the air-port, shows a black burn, singed grass and pieces of plane so small and splintered it's as if the aircraft evaporated. Two crew members, three flight attendants and twenty passengers were killed; nobody on board survived the impact. Dunham's ex-husband, and father to her daughter, was the captain on that plane. As an insider and a bereaved outsider, her sole purpose at the open day was to speak directly to the representatives of hundreds of airlines, gathered as they were in this room, to plead with them to stop using the word 'closure' – an insurance company word that means nothing. Nobody ever gets it. A crash never ends.

If closure is an unattainable point of reckoning, what does the presence of a body add to the new version of normal that is a living victim's life? What are we looking for, and how would a body help in finding it? It's a given we want the body back, and nobody questions it. But many struggle to look at it, some refuse. For some, religious belief places little significance in the body at all: the soul is gone, the empty vessel is less important than the spiritual idea of a person existing in another, better place. In a mass fatality, in wars, in natural or man-made disasters, millions are spent on returning bodies to families, whether whole or in pieces. What for? What does the presence of a body mean at a funeral if the coffin could be empty and no one would know but the pallbearers?

After General Franco's death in 1975, following nearly four decades of dictatorship, the Spanish government decided that instead of trawling through the crimes of the past – which historians have called the 'Spanish Holocaust', with a body count of hundreds of thousands – they would focus purely on the future of Spain. They voted to put in place a Pact of Forgetting, a kind of legislated amnesia, an amnesty law that meant nobody would be prosecuted for the mass suffering under Franco's rule, that the country would simply move on. Unlike Germany, they would not turn their own concentration camps into museums of remembrance or try officials before courts – the streets named in their honour would stay, the officials would remain in power, the slate would be wiped clean. It also meant that anyone who was thrown into a mass grave by Franco's soldiers would stay there; digging them up would be literally digging up the past, and it was forbidden by law to do so. Some of the surviving relatives of victims knew vaguely where the bodies were buried and flung flowers over walls or zip-tied them to roadside crash barriers. They were drawn to the places they believed their people were. Ascensión Mendieta was ninety-two when her father was finally located, in 2017, thrown into one of Spain's many mass graves after being killed by firing squad in 1939. When she heard the news that the grave was going to be exhumed (following a court case in Argentina, because crimes against humanity can be tried anywhere in the world, which helps if the state that committed them is suppressing cases by law) and that her father would be identified by DNA, she said, 'Now I can die happily. Because now I know I'll see him, even in a bone, or an ash.'

Mendieta died a year after her father was found in the cemetery where he was shot, where bullet holes were still visible on the walls. She had been campaigning all her life to get his bones back.

Seeing the body is a signpost, a mark on the trail of grief. The consoling tell the grieving that a person isn't really dead as long as you keep them alive in your mind, and this is true in more ways than the consoling person might intend. Without seeing your son's remains, or your dead infant's, they remain alive somehow, psychologically, in a way that all rational thought cannot defeat. In a plane crash, you could almost fool yourself that they are out there somewhere, that they survived the impact and washed up on a tropical island, that they are still manoeuvring rocks and logs to spell out SOS on the beach, waiting to be found. Without a body, you are caught in a twilight of death, without the complete darkness you need to reach acceptance.

'It's the limbo that people are in during this time that is so difficult,' says Mo. 'Not knowing where the body is. Not knowing if their loved one is going to be identified, even. Not knowing when they can have them back. It doesn't give those important staging posts that we have with normal death. A normal death might be a family member who you see getting ill before your eyes, who dies within hospital, and you're able to go to their funeral. And maybe they themselves speak to their family before they die. That's what's so difficult about homicides too: homicides are sudden and unexpected death. And in the same way that I did for homicide, I would tell a person, "Look, I'm going to do everything I can to try and find out what happened, to tell you what happened." This is the same type of drive, really. What's happened? How can I give you the truth? And sometimes that truth's pretty horrible. But the families want to know the truth, and we tell them everything.' You cannot give the families everything they want, but in recovering a body you can give them what they need to recover themselves.

The contents of Mo's go-bag are lined up on the carpet now, next to an empty brown leather carry-on. He's waiting for DNA results on victims in a plane crash. Tomorrow morning he'll fly to America to look in every body bag and make sure everything that is supposed to be there is there. On the blank Kenyon-branded labels in a sandwich bag on the floor, Mo will write the names of the identified people himself. He's been calling family members to tell them what he knows and talk them through the next steps – cremations, burials, it's all up to them. When the victim is released from the mortuary, Mo will be there. The casket will be the length and shape of a normal casket. Inside, just a small bag of pieces.

I want to know how all of this affects Mo, what it does to his psyche to see people piled in their mass graves, rotting in their body bags or sealed in pots. He says he feels no differently about death. 'Death is a part of living,' he says. 'That's one of the things that we do.' But his work has changed his priorities. You cannot see what he has seen and still think the same things matter. Prior to the tsunami in Sri Lanka, Mo says he was great at the bureaucracy that comes with working in the police service: the forms, the rules, the regulations. When he returned, it ceased to be important. 'It probably did a lot of damage to my career. Things just for the show, the gloss? Didn't care. I wasn't angry, I just wouldn't do it.'

His work has also given him a greater understanding of what people can handle emotionally, mentally, physically. Sri Lanka left one of his workers with PTSD, such that he'll likely never work again. 'I failed on that,' says Mo, bluntly and seriously. 'He worked non-stop for me without any days off for about three weeks. He was too fragile a person to have been sent in the first place.' There was a payout from the Home Office, in lieu of the aftercare he should have had. Kenyon is careful about which workers they take on a job, and there is mental-health support during the work and when it's over. Mo is currently arranging a debrief for the people on the Grenfell case. And after an experience in Kosovo – watching a volunteer on the exhumation team climb into the mass grave and retch every day for two weeks, refusing to quit – he knows there is a difference between wanting to go and actually being strong enough to do the job. Workers need to have the practical skills to assist, but they also need to be emotionally resilient: they cannot have suffered recent loss, they cannot be someone who has decided they are on a crusade to right wrongs they have experienced in their own lives.

He himself hasn't totally escaped the overwhelming nature of the job: in 2009, pre-Kenyon, he was deployed by the police to Brazil, to work on identifying the victims of the Air France 447 crash that left 228 dead. It was his first plane crash. His boss said he had to be back in time for his on-call shift in homicide, so he landed at Heathrow at 6 a.m. and drove straight to work, crashing his car on the way. 'My worlds had changed. My concentration wasn't on it. People need time to rest and recuperate after these.'

But Mo doesn't seem to rest. He says he's busy all the time. Unlike other people who worked with him in Sri Lanka – who never worked on another mass fatality, and organise an annual barbecue to check in with each other – Mo went to another big job, and then another. He keeps his shoes on during every flight, knows where his exits are and always watches the safety video to the end. And now he's here, working in an office where we're sitting just feet away from a warehouse holding the blackened possessions of people who burned to death in their beds. Like Nick Reynolds, the death mask sculptor, I wonder if everything would catch up with him if he ever sat still and thought about it. 'Now you're starting to sound like my wife,' he grins.

As I start putting my stuff in my bag and readying myself to leave, Mo asks me if anyone else I've spoken to has given me a good answer for why it is they do what they do. He's changed a bit since I arrived, he's less impish, he's looking reflective. We've been here for hours trying to figure out why he can do what he does; he insists that he's just 'a simple bloke' with nothing deeper to find, no big reason why he's ended up here. 'I'm pretty sure that under my superficial surface, all you'll find is more superficiality,' he keeps joking, drinking tea out of a mug that says 'PERFECT DAUGHTER'. But he tells me apropos of nothing that he has no unsolved murders. On his wall behind him is a framed quote from William Gladstone: *'Show me the manner in which a nation cares for its dead and I will measure with mathematical exactness, the tender mercy of its people, their respect for the law of the land and their loyalty to high ideals.'*

I tell him that over the past months, I've been given many reasons from people who think they have no reasons, but they all boil down to this: they are trying to help, and they are trying to do what they believe is right. They cannot reverse the situation and make people live again, but they can change how it is dealt with and give them dignity in death. I tell him about Terry in the Mayo Clinic, staying up late in the anatomy lab, waiting to swap the faces back even though no one would ever notice if he didn't. Mo nods silently, leans forward in his chair, the last mortuary padlock still between us. 'People deserve their identity, even after death. You know?'

The Horror

After a violent death, there is no US government agency that comes to clean up the blood, sparing property owners or family the sight of gore. When the body is in the van, the statements have been recorded, the fingerprints lifted and the police tape taken down, you are left with the mess and the quiet. 'Families, friends, nobody,' was who took care of it, the professional crime scene cleaner tells me. Neal Smither has a kind of California stoner, *that's-just-the-way-shit-is-man* quality to everything he says. Prior to his current job he had been really good at 'getting laid, smoking weed and sitting on the beach'. He's been cleaning death and crime scenes for the last twenty-two years, on call twenty-four hours a day. Now he sits by a stack of white napkins in a greasy diner wearing a crisp blue denim work shirt with a biohazard symbol embroidered on the breast pocket, and I ask him – because he would have seen it – what is the worst way to die.

'Unprepared.'

Most of the people he cleans up after were unprepared: didn't expect to be murdered, didn't expect to die in their sleep and decompose unnoticed until the rent was due, didn't expect life to go so wrong. Every couple of minutes, his phone beeps and vibrates with a new job. He ignores it. He is short, his hair neatly cut, his glasses smudge-free – he cleans them several times during our conversation. He asks the waitress for another stack of paper napkins, and she gives him maybe ten. Twice he will lean over and take more napkins to mop up invisible mess. He's loud and brash, but the sizzle off the grill obscures some of his words and he has to repeat them. People glance over shoulders. '*Decomposition*,' he says, louder. '*Brains*,' he repeats in the plural. '*Dildo*.'

Around us, chrome stools on black metal stems support the wide, blue-jeaned butts of Americans served by a waitress clutching a coffee pot in fingers extended by an inch of teal acrylic nail. A man with one eye and a limp leans on the Formica counter. An old couple wipe burger grease on each other's shirts – a side-effect of unconscious, reassuring back pats. There's a checkerboard floor, a jar of twenty-five-cent mint patties. A small TV plays nothing.

'There are three things that are almost always there at the scene of a murder,' he says, holding up fingers, casually knocking them down like faces in *Guess Who*. 'Porno or some kind of porn paraphernalia – from the tame to the, uh, you know. An inebriant of some kind, from gas, to chronic, to whatever your choice. And a weapon. The only thing that will really vary is the sexual aspect. Not everyone's leaving a dildo out on the dresser, but it's there somewhere. I'll find it.' I figure he's exaggerating, there can't possibly be a dildo at every murder scene. He gives me a look like I'm either underestimating or overestimating people. 'Life has stopped when we arrive,' he says. 'But they didn't clean up.'

Neal's company, Crime Scene Cleaners, Inc., is the line between looking normal and an atrocity exhibition – he's the reset button that allows you to put the house on the market after the murder or sell the impounded car at the police auction. Before companies like his existed, you personally got on your hands and knees and scrubbed the blood as best you could. Now, you can phone Neal. He will have a truck at your place within the hour. You can look the other way, go for coffee. Leave. When you return, it will look like nothing happened.

I'm talking to Neal partly because of what he does, but mostly because of how I found him. He markets his business the way anyone does: the internet. He has merch – hoodies, T-shirts, beanies – all bearing the same Crime Scene Cleaners, Inc. logo that he has tattooed on his forearm in a nest of skulls surrounded by the company's tagline: HOMICIDE – SUICIDE – *ACCIDENTAL DEATH*. Under the handle @crimescenecleanersinc on Instagram, where

he has almost half a million followers and his bio says, 'IF YOU
BITCH I BLOCK', he posts pictures of jobs before and after they have
been deep-cleaned. In idle scrolls I have seen the fine spray of
blood and brain reaching the upper limits of a room, hitting the
smoke detector and the light fitting after a shotgun suicide. Near
the crushed vehicle in a catastrophic car crash, shattered pieces of
skull, a brain stem on the tarmac. Teeth. When I found Neal, I was
doing what I've always done: I was looking for pictures of death on
the internet. I have followed his account for years.

I grew up as part of the generation that were the last to experience childhood without the internet, and the first to experience
it as teenagers. Back then, there were no safe searches: we could
explore anything the online world was offering, anything that we
could think of. Some went for pop stars and porno, others went
for death. Plug 'rotten.com' into the URL bar now and nothing
comes up, the website is defunct. But once upon a time it was
there, programmed in the stripped-back, basic html any teenager
taught themselves when starting a GeoCities website in the 1990s.
It was a collection of disease, violence, torture, death, human de-
pravity and cruelty in one grainy jpeg after another. There were the
famous, and there were the nobodies: the unidentified, the unidentifiable. There was *Saturday Night Live* star Chris Farley, overdosed
and purple-faced, dead on the floor of his apartment. Click.
A young blonde woman in the early stages of decomposition, her
green and yellow skin starting to slip. Click. A series of pictures sent
in by a policeman of a ninety-something-year-old man who had
died and inadvertently slow-cooked himself for two weeks with
the filament of a kettle submerged in the bathwater. Click. Another
comedian, Lenny Bruce, in the Celebrity Morgue offshoot site. In
September 1997, a year after the site began, its founder – a thirty-
year-old computer programmer for Apple and Netscape named
Thomas Dell, who ran the site anonymously under the pseudonym
Soylent – posted a photo of Princess Diana's corpse. Though the
photo was a fake, the sheer fact that he dared to publish it blew up
in the global press, and Rotten.com became infamous: a popular
destination for voyeurs, lawsuits, teenagers, me.

My impulse to look came from wanting to see the kind of everyday death that I could reckon with and understand, but all the internet could offer me was horror – I wasn't getting any further than I did when I was small, looking up at those Ripper crime scenes. I don't remember ever seeing anyone who died a natural death: they were mutilated, dismembered, exploded. They were a series of violent, unusual tragedies. Probably the closest to ordinary death was the mortuary photograph of Marilyn Monroe's blotchy face, comparatively serene. None of it ever felt like real death, or like something that even happened in my city. Plus, we were teenagers; we were immortal, even though my dead friend told me we were not.

I was ten when the website began, thirteen when I found it – about a year after Harriet's funeral. It was, to many of us who grew up in the early days of the internet (a/s/l?), formative. These are the things I was looking at in the one hour of dial-up I was allowed because more would cost another phone call. In another window I was chatting to kids from school on MSN Messenger, changing my display name to inside jokes and quotes from Coen brothers movies. The back of JFK's head, hair soaked with brain and blood, a click away from a chat about a boy. Teenage banality and horrific mortality side by side. 'The gruesome invites us to be either spectators or cowards, unable to look,' wrote Susan Sontag in her last published book before her death, *Regarding the Pain of Others*, an analysis of our response to images of horror. You picked a team: spectator or coward. It was compulsive, this need to see. It became something in itself. Once you had seen and could stand something terrible, you kept looking for the next worst thing. Through the struggling 56K modem, the pixels would load line by line, and your mind would race them to the bottom of the screen: were the things you saw worse or not as bad as you'd imagined? Sometimes the mess was so specific your mind could never have come up with it alone. You would never think a skull could crack like an egg, that brain could puddle like yolk. The teachers in the computer lab were not yet wise to us, pornography was not yet blocked.

You could see anything you wanted, and we went there to feel the buzz of unease and bravery that came with these images of death. Click enough and eventually you lost that buzz. You became numb.

It's this numbness I keep thinking about when I'm talking to Neal the crime scene cleaner. He's been the subject of a couple of documentaries and a reality TV show called *True Grime*; he's featured in an episode of *Mythbusters* and has done a string of YouTube guest spots. In reviews of his appearances, viewers often say he's cold-hearted – and sitting across from him, hearing about his career in sentences that could easily be voiceovers on late-night trash TV, I can see what they mean. Purely from his Instagram account I can see what they mean. But I wonder how much of that was already there, or whether it came with the job.

§

Like a lot of stoned twenty-something high-school dropouts watching *Pulp Fiction* in the mid-nineties, Neal had an epiphany about his life. Others went on to write derivative film scripts, Neal took a less obvious path. The scene that changed everything for him was when Harvey Keitel turns up as Winston Wolfe: he arrives in the early morning wearing a tuxedo, ready to solve the problem of John Travolta's Vincent Vega accidentally shooting Marvin's head off in the back of the car. 'You got a corpse in a car minus a head in the garage,' says the Wolf. 'Take me to it.' He directs Travolta and Samuel L. Jackson to shift the body to the trunk, take the cleaning products from under the sink and clean the car as fast as possible. He gets specific while Travolta and Jackson stand awkwardly in the kitchen in their blood-splattered suits and skinny black ties, Quentin Tarantino as Jimmie hovering in his dressing gown, dreading the imminent return of his wife. 'You gotta go in the back seat – scoop up all those little pieces of brain and skull, get it outta there. Wipe down the upholstery. Now, when it comes to upholstery, it don't need to be spick and span – you don't need to eat off it, just give it a good once over. What you need to take care of are the really messy parts – the pools of blood that have collected, you've gotta soak that shit up.' Travolta and Jackson trudged their way to the garage; Neal put his joint down and started a business.

He did some research into janitorial companies and found a couple of guys already on this bloody patch of turf, but they were so 'insultingly expensive' that he saw them as no threat. He took fifty bucks he couldn't afford, got himself a business licence and started hitting the pavement, shoving his flyers in the face of anyone who could use his services. He was doorstepping mortuaries and property management firms, and bribing cops in the Bay Area with doughnuts. 'It got to the point where the cops would see me coming, they'd hit the buzzer, I'd go right through. I'm inside the department; I'm going right down to homicide, I'm going to patrol, whatever. Back then, pre-9/11, you could do that. I'd bring Subway sandwiches and say, "Hey, motherfucker, when you gonna give me some work?" I just had great timing, and I was relentless. Every time you turned around, you were going to hear about me.' He says his grandmother, then in her eighties, got a volunteer gig at the Santa Cruz Police Department. From there she would write letters pretending she was a customer lauding his performance. She'd send letters to coroners, police sergeants, anyone they could think of who might have some sway in how a death scene disappears.

The diner we're in is the Red Onion on San Pablo Avenue in Richmond, north of San Francisco across the bay. 'This place is owned by a very stereotypical, old-school sergeant of Richmond Police Department,' says Neal, looking over his glasses at the Coca-Cola wallpaper and the ancient coffee machine. 'He was around when they'd club the shit out of you and nothing was gonna happen to them. He was one of the first guys I sold to.'

When the taxi dropped me off here an hour ago, the driver surveyed the place through squinted eyes and asked if I was sure. I got out, the car lingered. We both looked at the half-naked drugged man dragging a duvet through the parking lot of the Dollar Tree ('Everything's $1!') and past the drive-through Walgreens pharmacy. The small diner sat like an island in the middle of its own parking lot, looking like it teleported from the 1950s. Only months prior to this, a Swedish journalist named Kim Wall had been murdered on a submarine, her body dismembered and thrown in the sea between Denmark and Sweden. I didn't know her, but I knew her work, and at the time of her death we were writing for the same magazine. Had I found a man making his own submarine, I would have pitched that story too. I thought of her then, as I stood by the side of the road, about to meet a man whose job is to make murders disappear. The taxi driver looked up at me, and asked if I was absolutely sure I wanted to be left there. I nodded. 'OK, lady,' he said, and turned the car back onto the road without me.

'This is the place where shit goes down,' says Neal, motioning out the window, not making me feel any better about my choice. 'This is a magical market that I have control of. This is a very densely populated, small area. I've got millions of people available to me within a sixty-mile radius.' People, he says, are territorial animals. The more people you have, the more likely they're going to kill each other or themselves. Tensions rise in proximity.

This diner was where shit went down in April 2007 when the then-owner was shot in a botched robbery by four masked assailants. The detective in charge at the time described it to the *East Bay Times* as 'a takeover robbery, a real violent one'. They beat up a cook, cowed the other employees, and when Alfredo Figueroa appeared from the back office they shot him in the upper torso. They fled empty-handed. Figueroa died in the emergency room, his red Toyota 4Runner still parked days later in the cordoned-off parking lot. The men were never caught, and Captain Robert De La Campa of the El Cerrito Police Department told me that, as of 2019, the case remains under investigation. In the weeks following the incident, the family gave free burgers to anyone who donated $25 or more to the reward fund for information, cooked right here on the grill at the scene of the crime.

Neal has personal experience of cleaning a crime scene as a non-professional: the job fell to him aged twelve, when a neighbour committed suicide. The rifle bullet shot through his neighbour's head, broke the window, and splattered his brain up the side of the house where Neal was spending the summer with his grandparents. He took a steel scrubbing brush and a hose, and got to work. 'It was gross, but I didn't fucking care. I was more, "Whoa, that dude blew his fucking head off!" That tripped me out more. It just needed to be done. My grandparents couldn't do it, they were old. It was my job.' He got to it early, soon after the crack of the gun. Had he left it, he would have learned what he found out years later: that exploded brain dries like marble. It is still the hardest thing to clean.

If you can stay your gag reflex you can clean a death scene yourself, but hiring a professional depends on how much you care about the things you cannot see, and if you can afford to. Neal tells me to picture a house where a person has died and started to decompose. The body has been removed, so now you've just got the room with the mattress soaked in human fluid, the maggots, the stained floor. You remove the mattress, drench the scene in bleach, the place is visually spotless, and you think you're done. But you're not: you forgot about the microscopic feet of the flies. 'It took me a long time to realise the flies will walk in the door and track the mess all over everything,' he says. 'Unless you know that's happening, you don't even know where to look because you really can't see it until you get right up on the wall, or you touch the wall and the spot smears. You can pull the source, but it's *all over the fucking walls*.' His eyes widen. 'You gotta scrub *everything* down. You have to show the customers 'cause they don't believe you – and I wouldn't have either. I learned as I went, there wasn't an instruction manual. You know, fuck! Who knew?'

The majority of jobs Crime Scene Cleaners, Inc. take on – divvied up among the eight full-time staff, all men – are hoarding, rat infestations or blood-related. As to how that spills, it varies, and puddles of blood are another thing families underestimate. 'A bloody stain on the carpet is four times that size underneath the carpet. It's like an upside-down mushroom: you're looking at the end of the stem, underneath is the yummy cap. You have a plate-sized stain, but you're gonna have to cut four feet out of this carpet. Because blood separates. The white cells separate from the whatever the fuck it is, the plasma, and it makes a big, fat stain. It's the little shit like that they miss.'

At the end of each job, Neal will jump in the shower at the house and leave the scene clean and changed, because despite what Harvey Keitel's tuxedo might have you believe, the actual job is extreme manual labour. 'It's unglamorous and miserable,' Neal says. 'You're in a hazmat suit that you immediately start sweating in, you're soaked and you're in a fucking face mask. It's terrible.' I picture Terry back in the Mayo Clinic with his embalming fluid and sealed flooring, and ask Neal if the smell sticks with him despite the shower. 'Oh, yeah. But you don't really go in without a respirator on. The test is when you're done and you take your respirator off: can you smell it? If you can, there's a problem. You're not done. It's airborne, and it's not your airborne particulate, it's someone else's. You don't wanna ingest that, whether by breathing it or eating it or any other way of ingesting it.'

An eavesdropping customer turns mutely back to his milkshake.

§

As teenagers in the 1990s and early 2000s, looking at Rotten.com was deliberate. You had to mean it. It wasn't something you stumbled across on social media, where now you might see an image that has escaped the net of brand-protecting censorship, something you wish you could mentally erase. Back then, we had to go hunting. The website may be gone now, trapped in amber on the Wayback Machine, but similar ones have risen in its wake. The Crime Scene Cleaners, Inc. Instagram offers its own brand of horror for a new generation of death voyeurs: one that exists on a platform and in a timeline, with everything else. Sometimes, in the scroll, you can forget to consciously think about what it is you're seeing. Presented this way, slotted in among the rest of your curated life, there's a danger of the horror becoming mundane.

Images of death can be all around us, but we no longer process them as such because of their ubiquity. We are so accustomed to their presence, we become numb to them. You walk into a church and do not think anew that this is a tortured man, dead on a cross. The crucifixion is one of the most revisited moments in the history of art, but it is no longer shocking; it is a story you've heard again and again. You might have the image hanging around your neck but never notice it in the mirror: a public execution, a crime scene in twenty-four-carat gold. Through twelve years of Catholic school I was surrounded by the Stages of the Cross and Jesus's death. It was there in the elaborate stained-glass windows that blazed in the sun, it was there in the statues looming in the corner of every classroom, blood trickling out of his side. During Lent, when I was a child and this story was new, I knelt behind hard pews and listened to the priest tell us how many days Jesus lay in his tomb before he was resurrected, wondering what kind of state his corpse would be in, whether he was green when the stone rolled back. If he died on a Friday, what did he smell like on a Sunday? How hot does it get on Golgotha? Send your children to Catholic school. They'll have a great time.

Andy Warhol was brought up a Catholic and was obsessed with images of death. How could he not be – it's a religion built on them. According to those who were there at the time, Warhol's hang-up became particularly acute in the early 1960s when he was in his mid-thirties – my age. In June 1962, his friend and curator Henry Geldzahler handed him a copy of the *New York Mirror* over lunch. The headline screamed '129 DIE IN JET'; the text said the dead were from the art world. Warhol hand-painted the image of the plane wreck onto canvas. Two months later, Marilyn Monroe died. Only days after someone took the black-and-white photograph for the morgue file that would later turn up on the internet, Warhol made the first silkscreens of her famous, smiling face. The following months brought more additions to what he called his *Death and Disaster* series: suicide victims, car crashes, atomic bomb explosions, civil rights protesters attacked by dogs, two housewives poisoned by contaminated tins of tuna, and image after image of the electric chair in Sing Sing Correctional Facility thirty miles north of New York City. With every print and every repetition of the image, some duplicated over and over in a grid on the same canvas, Warhol got further and further away from the feeling the scene provoked, creating more distance between him and the reality – almost as if he had learned from church that repetition mutes the story.

I recognise this same effect in the Crime Scene Cleaners, Inc. Instagram account. Another grid, three across, dozens down – it's an amateur death and disaster series. They are images of tragedy, pain and violence, but taken in their hundreds, I am numb to them. It's Rotten.com all over again. 'The more you look at the same exact thing,' said Warhol, 'the more the meaning goes away, and the better and emptier you feel.'

It was always this series by Warhol that I lingered on as a teen-ager, in the pages of art books. He was interested in the same stuff I was. I never questioned why he might look for images of death, and it was only later that I realised our motivations were different: I was looking to understand death; he was trying to escape from it.

It never occurred to me that he was frightened. I thought he was just being provocative. He spoke of his fears to Geldzahler in phone calls late at night, small cries for help in the dark. 'Sometimes he would say that he was scared of dying if he went to sleep,' said Geldzahler. 'So he'd lie in bed and listen to his heart beat.' Warhol's brothers, John and Paul, believe that his crippling fear of death started with the death of their father, when Andy was thirteen. The body was brought home and laid out in the living room for three days. Andy hid under a bed, cried and begged his mother to let him stay at his aunt's house, and she – afraid that his nervous condition, Sydenham chorea, also known as St Vitus Dance, might come back – let him go.

Warhol never saw real death with his own eyes, he only saw what ran in the newspapers, through the lens of a photographer. At thirteen he – unlike me – had been given the option to see death up close, and he said no. It wasn't until the seventies, on the other side of Valerie Solanas's near-fatal bullet, that he started exploring his own mortality in self-portraits and skulls. But his fear remained throughout his life: Warhol never went to funerals or wakes, refusing to attend even his mother's burial in 1972. He was a victim of images that held the power to haunt him, and through his art he tried to fight against that power, rather than seize real-life opportunities to see death as anything other than horrifying. His beautiful avoidance behaviour hangs in galleries around the world.

'Ever since cameras were invented in 1839, photography has kept company with death,' wrote Sontag. The reasons for taking these photographs are numerous, as varied as the motivations of the people who look. Victorians mounted cameras on tripods to take pictures of the dying and the dead – sometimes the only photograph they would ever have of their child, nestled there in the thick fabric that concealed a mother holding her dead baby, or maybe it was laid out in its tiny coffin, devastated parents posed stiffly beside it while they waited for the exposure. Then there were the crime scene and autopsy photos, taken for police purposes, like the ones in 1888 of the five dead women that I knew so well: Polly Nichols, Annie Chapman, Elizabeth Stride, Catherine Eddowes, Mary Kelly. Decades later, a photographer called Weegee (real name Arthur Fellig) helped sell newspapers using death as a sensationalist attraction, recording the violence of the 1930s: the end of the Depression, the repeal of Prohibition and the governmental crackdown on organised crime that resulted in a surge of murders across New York City. He never photographed the action, just the immediate aftermath – thanks to his police radio (he was the only freelance newspaper photographer with a permit to have one) he'd get there in time to snap the body in the pool of blood and the gangster's hat upturned on the pavement before the white sheet came down. His photographs would be splashed across the front pages: hundreds of bodies, hundreds of stories, all of them ripped out and pinned to the walls of his dingy studio apartment across the road from the New York City Police Department, like trophies. Victims lined the room. 'Murder,' he said, 'is my business.'

Far apart from the ethically shaky world of tabloid newspapers, photojournalism serves a vital role in documentary proof, where eyesight and testimony are fallible. In 1945, Margaret Bourke-White – the first American female war photojournalist and the first woman allowed to work in combat zones – travelled through a

collapsing Germany with General Patton's Third Army. Her photos
of Nazi atrocities, taken when she would have been forty years
old, are unflinching, important records that she was only able
to mentally process later, in the dark room. 'I kept telling myself that I would believe the indescribably horrible sight in the
courtyard before me only when I had a chance to look at my own
photographs,' she wrote in her memoir the following year, of the
scenes at Buchenwald. 'Using the camera was almost a relief; it
interposed a slight barrier between myself and the white horror in
front of me.' Her photographs, published in LIFE magazine, were
some of the first reports to show the reality of the death camps to
a largely disbelieving public.

A photojournalist sits on the line between record and action: their
work is essential for the world to know what's happening, but it can
come at great personal cost. Kevin Carter won the Pulitzer prize
for his 1993 photograph of a starving, collapsed child in Sudan
being watched over by a vulture. When it ran in the paper, readers
wrote in to the New York Times wanting to know what had happened
to her, wanting to know if the photographer had helped. Days later,
the paper ran a notice saying the vulture was shooed away and the
child continued her journey, though it was not known if she made
it to the food tent. Three months after winning the Pulitzer, at
the age of thirty-three, Carter gassed himself in his pickup truck,
leaving a note behind. It said, in part, 'I am haunted by the vivid
memories of killings & corpses & anger & pain ... of starving
or wounded children, of trigger-happy madmen, often police, of
killer executioners.'

As a viewer of images of death, the crucial element is context: we need to know what happened or they float loose in our
memories as unmoored horror, the effects of which might be ac-
cumulative fear or numbness, depending on who you are. Pictures
of crime scenes, as they appear on Neal's Instagram, are none of
the above. They are not a call to arms, and they are not a story
that elicits empathy or a deeper understanding. They don't even
sell newspapers. They are just meaningless gore. Mostly this is because we do not know the story at all: though he is usually given

an explanation by police dispatch as a way of estimating the length of the job, Neal says the captions he writes are never the actual truth – he'll change the narrative to something unrelated as a way of masking identities, though occasional family members still find the posts and rage at him in the comments. There isn't really a point to these images at all, other than voyeurism and the promotion of his business, but it's more of a performance piece than a display of what your money can buy. He began the account to show people what his job is like, and though he doesn't actually get many customers through the feed, the vague nature of the posts creates a buzz around the business: in the comments, in the absence of details, followers construct a narrative of their own, piecing together things glimpsed through the partially obscured window that Neal has allowed them into these private death scenes.

The only part of the story we know to be true is that the crime scene cleaner is arriving at scenes that have already played out, the crime already committed, the wrist already slit – the story he cannot change. I wonder if any of this weighs on him. It doesn't appear to. 'I think it's none of my business, really,' he says. I ask about images that stick in his mind, and Neal struggles to find one. A toddler's footprints down a hallway in her parents' blood, maybe. But mostly nothing. 'Everyone starts out wanting to know the stories – your first fifty jobs or so – and then you don't care, you don't even see it,' he says. 'You've forgotten it, in most cases, by the time you leave the house.'

Towards the end of her analysis of the effect horrific images have on us, Sontag wrote that 'compassion is an unstable emotion. It needs to be translated into action, or it withers ... One starts to get bored,' she says, 'cynical, apathetic.' Whether or not the unstable emotion of compassion was ever there, cynicism now appears to reign supreme in Neal. It is there in the way he talks about his work, to me, in the diner. It is there in the blunt captions on photographs he hashtags '#p4d': pray for death, because death equals cash (murder is his business too). Some of the things he says to me I have heard almost verbatim in other places, on TV, on YouTube. 'If I wasn't out there pissing everyone off on TV and giving great soundbites, the company wouldn't be near where it's at now,' he says. It's all part of the performance of being the internet's crime scene cleaner. I am struggling to have any real sense of how he feels about anything, or even how I feel about Neal. I have been another audience to a well-practised show, polished until it shines.

But there are some moments where I get flashes of something true.

Neal doesn't go out on cleaning jobs much any more. His staff send him the photographs to post online. He's fifty now, and says his imperfect eyesight lessens his ability to get the microscopic fly prints off the walls, but mostly he stays out of it because he can no longer hide his feelings. 'I'm not sympathetic to the customer any more, and I think that probably reflects more than I want it to. They just *disgust* me,' he says. 'I don't explicitly tell them I think they're assholes, but they can feel it.'

It's this disgust for the customer that keeps coming up – towards both their attitude and their filthy houses. It wasn't always present, but after twenty-two years of cleaning up horror and tragedy, he sees only the worst of us. 'I think everyone's just kind of opportunistic, and looking out for themselves,' says Neal, before telling me there is no such thing as loyalty. In cases where a person has died and been left undiscovered for months, families will turn up to go through the stuff in the house, trawling it for treasure they can sell. 'I'm cleaning and they're picking through the drawers, looking for items that they can keep like it's their birthright. I *hate* that.'

Neal went into this job with cold, capitalist intentions and, to him, this job is still just cleaning and money. 'I'm not here to be your friend, I'm not here to be your shrink,' he says, the last bites of his burger disappearing. 'I'm your janitor, you know? What do you care what I think of you?' In his work, he doesn't have any sense of making the world a better place or giving the dead person their dignity; his job is to remove all traces of a person from the scene, to literally dehumanise the situation in order to make the house sellable for the third cousin going through the drawers in the other room. But they are both in the house for the same reason, and maybe that's the root of Neal's disgust. They are the vultures, and they are paying him.

He tells me he has a place in Idaho where he and his wife are going to retire, a clean oasis where he will go off the grid and leave all the murders, suicides, rats and forgotten people behind. He grabs his phone, swipes the dozens of job notifications away and shows me a countdown clock, the numbers ticking over second by second. 'The day I go black is 1,542 days from now. Four years and two months and twenty days.' He can't wait to get there. 'That's where I'm dying,' he says. He's prepared: he has all of his affairs in order, and before he can't physically do it any more, he wants to hike up into the mountains and get eaten by a bear. He doesn't want to end up as someone else's cleaning job.

'Are you afraid of death?' I ask.

'Yeah. I don't wanna die.'

He asks if we're done, picks his keys up off the table and talks to the staff on the way out. The waitress leans on the counter, order pad tucked into a cocked hand at her waist, asks him if he's busy. He says he's always busy. His phone pings again. He tells me to wait for my ride inside the diner, says it's not safe out there. I watch him drive off in his immaculate Ram pickup truck, spotless and white, glinting in the sun; every other car in sight matte with dirt, absorbing light like black holes. His number plate says HMOGLBN. Instagram tells me he recently bought a new truck for an employee. It says BLUDBBL.

I tuck myself back into the booth and wait for a cab to pick me up. I take out my phone and I scroll. There, nestled between the dogs and selfies and houseplants in rose-gold pots, are fresh crime scenes.

Dining with the Executioner

On 27 February 2017, it was announced that the state of Arkansas was going to rush through the execution of eight prisoners in the space of eleven days. It was a pace unseen in recent American history – Arkansas itself had not carried out even a single execution in twelve years. Their reasoning was that their limited supply of midazolam, one of three drugs used in the state's lethal-injection protocol, was approaching its use-by date and so, by extension, were these eight men. (Arkansas is no stranger to newsworthy death penalty decisions: this is the same state that, in 1992, saw then-governor Bill Clinton rush home from his presidential campaign trail to witness the execution of Ricky Ray Rector, a man so mentally impaired by a self-inflicted gunshot wound to the head that he saved his last meal dessert, a slice of pecan pie, for after his execution. Refusing to pardon the man was a PR move on Clinton's part. He wanted to look less soft.)

In a letter dated 28 March 2017, signed by twenty-three former death row staff from across the nation, they pleaded with Governor Asa Hutchinson:

'We believe that performing so many executions in so little time will impose extraordinary and unnecessary stress and trauma on the staff responsible for carrying out the executions … Even under less demanding circumstances, carrying out an execution can take a severe toll on corrections officers' well-being. For those of us who have participated in or overseen executions, we have directly experienced the psychological challenges of the experience and its aftermath. Others of us have witnessed this same strain in our colleagues. The paradoxical nature of corrections officers' roles in an execution often goes unnoticed: the officers who have dedicated their professional life to protecting the safety and wellbeing of prisoners are asked to participate in the execution of a person under their care.'

The letter to Governor Hutchinson had little effect; within a month of it being sent, four men were executed and the other four had been given stays unrelated to its attempted intervention. Even the lesser number of four executions in a week, in one facility, stands alone in the modern history of American capital punishment.

I found Jerry Givens's name at the bottom of this letter, attached to the news story that I had come across that morning. In the long list of signatories – wardens, captains, a chaplain – he was the only one listed as 'executioner'. Modern-day executioners are anonymous, or at least they are to us; their identities are kept from newspaper reports, and their jobs are carried out behind prison walls. So why was an executioner not only publicly naming himself, but signing this letter about trauma? What happened?

To me, executioners were always a kind of satellite moon to the death workers I was interested in – they were not one of their group, but they existed within their orbit as other invisible people who work in the death trade. But an executioner is not the crime scene cleaner, scrubbing away the aftermath of something he did not do and cannot change. They are not the mortuary worker in the funeral home receiving the already dead body and writing the name on the refrigerator door. The executioner is there at the transition from life to death; they are the cause of it, in the most basic practical sense – the final part of a machine that carries out the directives of the government and the court, doing the work that others would rightly balk at. What is it like to walk into that room, strap a person into an electric chair and flip the switch? To turn a living, healthy person into a corpse and then go home, having done your job, having ended a human life? Why would a person take that job and keep it?

Here, in this letter, was an executioner trying to save another execution team from whatever it was he experienced. Maybe he would talk to me, and tell me how he felt; it seemed he now had a reason to do just that. I wanted to know how someone who has ended lives by planned, state-sanctioned murder deals with the psychological pressure of that fact. What does death mean to him if it is just another tier of punishment that can be handed down in a court of law? Does he fear death more or less now that he has seen not only the bodies, but the moment it happens?

This is not what I tell the woman at the hotel check-in desk as she's plugging my credit card number into the system, when she pauses to say with all the honesty of someone who is tired and wants to go home, 'My God. Why are you in Richmond, Virginia?'

§

I've been trying to pin Jerry down for a year and every time I ask him for a good day to meet he casually says to just let him know the week before I get into town. It's a vague plan to fly around the world for, but I've probably done stupider things. So I wangle some other magazine work in America, the idea being that if he doesn't turn up the trip isn't a total bust, and organise the itinerary so that Virginia is on the way — despite the fact that Virginia, located where it is, is hardly on the way to anywhere I'm going.

On the day Jerry and I have agreed to meet, my boyfriend, Clint, and I drive the 250 miles down from Philadelphia in a shitty Nissan rental. I've convinced him to come with me because this trip is a little complicated to rely on cabs for, and while it's a part of my job to talk to people in strange places — basements, remote film sets, small Scottish towns with one cab driver who is always in the shower when you call — after the crime scene cleaner, I've finally had enough of sitting and watching the dot of a car move slowly on an app towards me while I worry about patchy signal being the only thing between me and everything falling apart. Also, I'm meeting an actual executioner in a place he hasn't yet specified, in a part of America where I know nobody — I'll be honest, I feel weird about that. Not that I'm saying you should bring an English comedian with you if you fear for your life, but they are traditionally better at driving long distances in shitty cars.

It's late afternoon in January. It's dark. We're aiming for Richmond but we don't know where exactly, and Jerry calls to ask where we are. We're stuffing our faces with crisps in an empty petrol station wondering just how loose this plan can get. We're also wondering how long two people can survive on things they find in petrol stations, two people who wouldn't have to live like this if whoever had done the itinerary factored in stopping for lunch. The car smells like old pizza and so do we. Jerry tells me to meet him at the school. He'll be out front. Which school? He emails me the address. It's a school in the suburbs – why does an executioner want to meet me there, hours after class has finished? We drive some more, following the crumbs across the world as he drops them. The licence plates on the vehicles in front of us say 'Virginia is for lovers', all of them manufactured by inmates at a prison shop west of the city centre.

It's 7 p.m. We drive down a quiet street where the streetlights don't work so well but the headlights of the car briefly illuminate a 'BLACK LIVES MATTER' banner hung from the roof of a community hall. We pull up by Armstrong High School, barely lit outside bar the lights from the lobby pooling out on the pavement. There's nobody around except for the silhouette of a guy smoking by his car. He doesn't react to our arrival, so I assume he isn't Jerry. We grab our bags and walk over to the school entrance. Having travelled so far in a car with one working windscreen wiper and a bumper we reattached with a zip tie, I'm sort of resigned to whatever absurdity awaits us. I have no idea what to expect from someone who served as the state's executioner for seventeen years.

I squint through the glass doors. I can see security guards and metal detectors – that surreal American high-school scene – and a few steps up, on the mezzanine, I can see a black man in his sixties, with glasses and a white beard, bending down so he can peer through the security gates at our faces. He grins and warmly waves us in. Aside from the few people here, it's still, as far as I can tell, an empty school. Even the hallways off the lobby are dark.

'They with you, Jerry?' asks one of the guards.

'Yeah, they are. All the way from London!' He chuckles. He has a slow, Southern way of speaking, the kind of deep voice you want to hear on the radio late at night.

The guards go through our bags, pat us down for guns and knives. 'We're from England,' I say awkwardly. 'We've got nothing.' They smile and wave us through. Jerry gives me a hug and says thanks for coming, he's glad we made it. 'We're going to go and watch a basketball game,' he says. 'You like basketball?'

I didn't expect a basketball game.

We walk through the dim halls, Jerry in his tan trousers and navy jacket, a slight limp from recent knee surgery. We give $14 to a man at a desk with a little petty-cash lunch box and he hands us a couple of ticket stubs, tells us to enjoy the game. 'They with you, Jerry?' he asks.

'Yeah, they with me,' he smiles, and limps on ahead.

Jerry pushes open the double doors to the high-school gym and the light is dazzling. It smells of fresh varnish and sweat, and the squeaks of shoes on the slick floor deafen. It's the Wildcats versus the Hawks. We've arrived in time for the third quarter, and Jerry takes a seat in the bleachers, waving at people as he passes. The school principal stands grinning in his suit and purple tie by the home basket. A tiny girl with cornrows hugs her brother's enormous white Nikes in her lap.

Clint and I squeeze in next to him, shoulders hunched in the way that trees grow in a forest so their canopies don't touch, and Jerry tells me, in words that get lost occasionally in the squeaks and cheers, that he went to this school himself in 1967; when it opened in the 1870s, it was the first school to teach African Americans in Virginia. He tells me that for the last thirty years he's been mentoring the kids here; he'd come after work, still wearing his prison uniform, and let them ask him anything they wanted about prison life while kicking the ball around at football practice. 'It gave me some opportunity to steer these kids in the right direction, because a lot of them would go out and do the same thing that their parents did, what their friends did, and they'd end up on Spring Street. That's where the jail was,' he says. 'That's where they'd execute people.'

'Travel!' shouts a coach.

Someone blows a whistle.

§

Back in 1974, when Jerry first got his job as a correctional officer at the state penitentiary, there was no death penalty in Virginia – there was no death penalty in the country at all. The United States was in the midst of a brief nationwide moratorium on capital punishment, bookended by two court cases. *Furman v. Georgia*, in 1972, invalidated all death penalty sentences, arguing that they were cruel and unusual, and reduced them to life imprisonment while the country figured out a way of applying them with more consistency and with (supposedly) less racial discrimination. Statutes across the country were amended to meet Supreme Court guidelines, and in 1976, *Gregg v. Georgia* reopened the doors of the country's death chambers.

Virginia – one of the thirteen original colonies, and home to founding father Thomas Jefferson's Charlottesville plantation – has a long history of execution. What is generally agreed to be the first American execution was carried out there in Jamestown, by firing squad, ending the life of Captain George Kendall in 1608 for allegedly plotting to betray the British to the Spanish. But in 1977, when Jerry's supervisor offered him a role on the 'death team', Virginia's death row was empty. They hadn't executed anyone there since 1962.

Jerry was just twenty-four years old at the time. If you had asked him then, he would have said he was pro-capital punishment – take a life and your life should be taken. He says he remembered being at a party when he was fourteen, seeing someone walk into the house and shoot dead a girl he'd been too nervous to talk to. The injustice of it had stuck in his mind. So he took the job, which he was told would come with a cash bonus for each execution carried out. When I ask him how many dollars an executioner would get per job, he says he doesn't know; he never asked.

He never accepted any extra payment for what he did, because it would have changed the purpose of his being there. 'My job was *saving* lives,' he says. 'You know how many times I risked my life saving another inmate's life, or an officer's life?'

'In fights?'

'Mm-hmm. Stabbing and everything, inside the institution.'

Jerry didn't know who else the supervisor had asked, but after he accepted the role he and those eight other guys met in the prison basement one night to swear anonymity. Nobody outside the death team knew who was on it. Jerry didn't even tell his wife – and he wouldn't, for the entire time he held the position.

Every death penalty state in the country has their own way of appointing an executioner – before the moratorium, some executioners were not even prison staff but worked as freelance 'electricians' called in just for the purpose of throwing the switch. In the state of New York, some were known to the public by name – one received death threats, one had his house bombed. Some made lots of money off it, going from state to state, collecting a check for each life ended. Others worked anonymously: one would change the plates on his car in his garage before he left in the middle of the night for the long drive to Sing Sing, so that he could not be identified or traced. The man who operated Florida's electric chair would already be wearing a hood when the car picked him up at 5 a.m. to take him to the death house – it stayed on until he walked back through his front door. When the moratorium ended, fresh teams were formed across the country (Florida was less covert than most and put out an ad for the job in the paper; they received twenty applications). The new teams learned how to use whatever equipment was left behind by the old ones: gas chambers, electric chairs, nooses and guns.

Virginia's original electric chair, constructed by inmates in 1908 from an old oak tree, was unpacked and reassembled (Jesus was a carpenter too, and the irony of creating the weapon of your own destruction was not lost on my teenage self – or Nick Cave). In 1982, they prepared it for use on Frank James Coppola – a thirty-eight-year-old former police officer who had bound a woman with the cord from a Venetian blind during a robbery, slammed her head repeatedly into the floor until she was dead, then fled with $3,100 in cash, plus jewellery. Jerry was only the alternate executioner that night. It would not be him who pressed the button for the first time in twenty years – someone else on the team had that job.

There was no media present to report what happened in that room. News items on executions tend to be unreliable and inconsistent anyway – dramatised and exaggerated both ways, bent to the newspaper's politics. No corrections officials released details of the execution either. But according to one account by an attorney who was present as a witness, as a representative to the General Assembly of Virginia, it did not go well. The antiquated machinery set Coppola's leg alight; smoke rose to the ceiling and filled the chamber with a foggy haze. During the second and final fifty-five-second jolt of electricity, the attorney heard a sizzling that he described as sounding 'like cooking flesh'.

Coppola was not the first to experience a botched electrical execution: that wired crown goes to William Kemmler in 1890, New York – an alcoholic who had murdered his common-law wife in a drunken argument, hitting her twenty-five times in the head with a hatchet. He was the first to be executed by electrical current, if we don't count the old horse they tested the voltage on.

He was also the first to demonstrate that the human skull is a poor conductor of electricity, as is skin: from the autopsy report printed in the New York Times the day after his execution, when the burned skin on his back was removed, the pathologist described his spinal muscles as looking like 'overcooked beef'. Sweat, however, is an excellent conductor – being essentially salt water and therefore containing more conductive ions than pure water – and most people being walked to a death chamber and strapped into an electric chair will drench themselves in it. Execution teams learned to soak the sponge in saline solution and place it on the condemned person's shaved head, between the skin and the helmet. Jerry tells me that many modern-day botched executions

are as a result of prisons using synthetic sponges – instead of natural ones – which set the head alight.

Two years after the Virginia death team executed Coppola,
Linwood Earl Briley sat in that same oak chair. He and his
two brothers were responsible for a seven-month robbery and
murder spree across the city of Richmond, in 1979, that officially left eleven people dead, though investigators suspected
them of killing almost twice that. The lead executioner called
in sick that day, so Jerry took the role – strapping the man in,
wetting the sponge and placing it on his shaven head, standing
behind a curtain and pushing the button that would send the
current through his body and stop his heart. Was the previous
executioner actually ill, or could he not face the death chamber
after what had happened to Coppola, knowing it was his finger
that started it all? I can't ask him – Jerry won't say who it was.
He still respects the promise of anonymity he made that night
in the basement when he was twenty-four. At any rate, that
person was never the lead executioner again. Of the 113 people
killed in the Virginia death chamber since its reopening, the
next sixty-two of them were Jerry's – twenty-five by electric
chair, and thirty-seven by lethal injection.

§

We follow the tail-lights of Jerry's Kia to Red Lobster for dinner,
another brightly lit American chain island in a car-park ocean.
Walk through the front doors and before you're shown a table, you
meet the inmates: a tank of condemned lobsters awaiting execution, little rubber handcuffs around their immovable claws, walls
of cloudy Perspex dividing up their prison cells. They stare up at
us, unblinking.

'Pick one,' says Jerry, grinning.

I stand there, Caligula in a cagoule, choosing which one is going
to die. They crawl over each other to get a better look at us.

There's a Charles Addams cartoon I think about sometimes: two half-dressed executioners in a brick alcove, a kind of
pre-beheading dressing room, wearing their hoods and cloaks,

pulling on their long black gloves. One of them is leaning on his axe saying to the other, 'The way I see it, if we don't do it, someone else will.' It pops into my mind now. Someone else has marked these lobsters for death, and if I don't pick one someone else will. Even so, I can't do it. I can't press the button on a lobster's life. I tell Jerry I'm going to order something else and he laughs. Clint and I stare into the tank while he wanders off and waves to the staff. They know him here too. He's halfway to the table and I'm still weighing my guilt next to the four-pound crustaceans.

I've barely slid into the booth when he starts telling me that God put him in the position to kill people, so if I'm here to find out why he was chosen for the job, I'll have to speak to God directly. 'He had his reasons. I didn't ask why, I just took on that position. I didn't put myself in that. You think, at twenty-four years old ... and *a black man* to do this?' He looks incredulous. 'But –' he shrugs – 'it was gonna be done regardless if I did it or not. Because the state can do it.' There's that Charles Addams cartoon again. I glance back at the lobsters. He picks up his menu and says he doesn't know about us, but he's going to go for something called the Ultimate Feast.

Paul Friedland writes in his book *Seeing Justice Done: The Age of Spectacular Capital Punishment in France* that this image we have of an executioner as an agent of the law, someone whose job it is to carry out a sentence handed down from above, is a relatively modern idea purposely put in place by Enlightenment reformers who were trying to construct a different kind of penal system – one that was rational and bureaucratic, one that dispersed responsibility, and therefore blame, among many cogs in a vast system. Prior to this, in France at least, the executioner was considered an extraordinary being, an outcast, a universally reviled person 'whose touch was so profane that he could not come into contact with other people or objects without profoundly altering them'. They lived on the edges of towns and married within their kind. The role of executioner was usually one that was inherited: you were damned by having executioners' blood run in your veins, as if you yourself had let the blade of the guillotine fall. When executioners died, they were buried in a separate section of the cemetery, for fear that their presence – alive, dead, there was no difference – would contaminate the general population. They were untouchables, in the literal sense, given long-handled spoons with which to take produce from market stalls, and wore special insignia so that no one might mistake them 'for someone honourable'. 'Throughout the early modern period, and indeed through the Revolution as well,' writes Friedland, 'one of the most effective means of impugning someone's moral character was to insinuate that they had been seen dining with the executioner.' Jerry politely signalled to the waiter that we were ready for him to take our order.

'Did the prisoners ever know you were the guy pressing the button?' I ask. Incarcerated men have a lot of time to think. I imagine they would have their theories about the wardens and captains – being an executioner is not a full-time job.

'Uh-uh,' he says, shaking his head. 'Some of them would guess. They'd get to the end and go, "I'm willing to bet it's you, Givens, that's pulling that switch." I said, "No bud, it ain't me." I'm not gonna sit there and tell them that I am! So I laughed it off. "It ain't me, bud. It ain't me."'

Executions, during Jerry's time, happened at 11 p.m. – as late as possible to allow for last-minute appeals, with a spare hour in case there was a fault with the equipment (miss the midnight deadline and you have to wait for the courts to hand down a new date of execution). Jerry had many waking hours to think about it, watching the clock tick down to either a stay or an order, a life or a death. His job was preparation, for both the inmate and himself.

'I prepared a guy for his next phase of life,' says Jerry, forking a deep-fried shrimp as the plate is slid in front of him. 'I don't know where he was going, so it's between him and his maker, between him and God. But my thing is to get you ready. How do you prepare yourself to be killed? I studied him, I talked to him, I prayed with him. Because this is his last everything.'

While he was inside helping the condemned to put their affairs in order, both spiritual and practical, death penalty advocates would gather outside the prison, selling T-shirts, holding banners, celebrating. Abolitionists would crowd around their candles nearby for a silent vigil. To the condemned man, the hours felt like minutes. To the executioner, the seconds dragged as if the hands of the clock were stuck. How do you psychologically prepare yourself for ending the life of someone you've been caring for as a warden?

'I blocked everything out,' he says. 'I focused on what I had to do. I don't talk to nobody. I don't even look in the mirror, because I don't want to see myself as the executioner.'

A cheery waiter comes by and puts some drinks down while I picture a man avoiding himself in the mirror. 'This whole time, with your wife not knowing – didn't you feel like you wanted to tell her?'

'No, because if you was my wife, and you knew I had an execution, then whatever stresses I'm going through you're going to go through too. You're going to feel for me. So I never put that on her.'

§

Every state is different, but typically the identity of the executioner is kept vague not only to the inmate and the witnesses but to the death penalty team itself, so everybody feels that it is nothing they did on their own. Sometimes there are two switches pressed simultaneously and the machine decides which button will be live, then automatically deletes the record, so no one can be certain they were the one who dealt the blow – either electrical or chemical. Put enough robotics between you and the act and you can fool yourself into believing it barely happened, like drone strikes. Other times, it's the person themselves who diffuses the responsibility: Lewis E. Lawes, a warden at Sing Sing from 1920 to 1941, directed the execution of more than 200 men and women in the electric chair but looked away when the switch was flicked, allowing him to claim that he had never seen an execution. But despite the fact that Jerry's team, like all death teams, split up their tasks among themselves so that no one person shouldered the burden alone, it was only Jerry who pressed the button on the control panel. It was only Jerry who watched the lethal chemicals travel from the syringe in his own hand, down the tube and into the vein of the man strapped to the gurney. But even with this certainty, or maybe because of it, he has managed to place a block between himself and the act of killing someone: God.

Jerry believed the death wasn't truly an end because there was an afterlife – and so did many of the inmates, after enough years on death row. Even the former atheists needed something to look forward to, some higher power to ask for forgiveness when the state would not give it to them. They needed some hope of an intervention, a last-minute reprieve, some force that might make the phone on the wall of the death chamber ring – another irony, looking for clemency from the same guy who permitted his only son to be killed by way of state execution. It seems that everyone on death row, from the prisoners to the wardens, to the politicians and judges who refused the pardons, shifted the weight of responsibility onto God. I've always been wary of anyone using religion as a shield, or a proxy; to me, it says they're choosing not to think too deeply on whatever it is they're doing because it doesn't matter, it's someone else doing it. They're only following orders from above. In a place like Virginia's death house, God is the soft focus everyone puts on the scene.

But for Jerry, all of this is a retrospective rewrite – a first draft with plot holes and contradictions. He tells me that God put him in that position, and he was doing God's work. He says he talks to God every day, but when I ask when that conversation started, the date he gives me is years after he left the job. The timeline doesn't fit – he wasn't talking to God when he was in that death chamber, he wasn't talking to anyone. I cannot, no matter how many times I prod or rephrase the question, get into his headspace in those early executions: what he was thinking as he put on his pressed uniform, as he avoided himself in the mirror and kissed his wife goodbye. Maybe he can't either; the body tucks our trauma away in dark spaces, we build narratives with blank spots to save ourselves.

But whether you shift the blame onto God, a judge or a jury, when a person is executed by the state, the official manner of death on their certificate reads 'homicide'. Whether you be-lieve it is a fitting and fair punishment for the horrific crimes committed, 'the machinery of death cannot run without human hands to turn the dials' wrote David R. Dow, founder of Texas's oldest innocence project, and those hands were Jerry's; he has to live with them. I can tell he's getting frustrated with me for pointing this out, over and over, while the waiter leans over to take our empties.

'Listen,' he says, cutlery in his fists, resting on the edge of the table. He's not angry, he's chuckling at the obviousness of it all, at the naivety of me. 'I didn't kill nobody for myself,' he smiles se-renely. 'You was gonna be killed anyway. I was just in a position to press that button. I'm the last resolve, I'm the last one that will take responsibility for what you did. You understand? You knew exactly what you were getting into, when you went out and you murdered this person. You forfeit your life. You made a bad choice. There was a consequence. It's *suicide*, sweetheart. It is.'

We look at each other over the ruin of napkins and fish and I say nothing. I don't know what to say. He's spent years – within prison walls and without – building up this mental scaffolding that allows him to carry on without collapsing, and who am I to try to pull it down? Joan Didion wrote in *The White Album*, 'We tell ourselves stories in order to live … We look for the sermon in the suicide, for the social or moral lesson in the murder of five. We interpret what we see, select the most workable of the multiple choices.' Even the death squad leaders in the 1965 Indonesian genocide told themselves they were cool Hollywood gangsters, like James Cagney, as they garrotted countless numbers on rooftops bathed in blood. Someone in the booth next to us laughs. The bland pop ballads are punctuated by bells from the kitchen. More than any-thing, Jerry is likeable and sweet – the way he is with the kids at the school, the way he is with the waiting staff who know him as a regular and the way he is with me. I just can't picture him being the executioner at all.

'But,' I start, 'didn't you think, the first time you had to take a life, I *can't do this*? Or did you know you would be capable of—'

'Listen,' he says, picking up the bread basket and dumping the last two cheese biscuits onto the table. 'Sweetheart. You losing it. I didn't take his life. He took his own life. This the inmate —' he waggles his phone — 'this the river.' He holds up the empty bread basket and plonks it back down. 'If you do wrong, you're going to fall into this river and die.' He *choo-choos* the bread basket across the table between the bottles of beer and iced tea, parting a sea of napkins. 'You're gonna do wrong?' He throws his phone in the bread basket. 'You die. I'm here, behind this big building —' he moves the ketchup bottle into play — 'with a button. I haven't pushed it, I've never used it. Don't have to use it. Make right choices, you don't come past me — you go right by me.' He pushes the bread basket, it sails on past the sticky bottle. 'Don't give me a chance to use that button. Do you hear what I'm saying? Don't put the blame on me. It's nothing that I do. I'm not gonna lose no sleep over it.'

I say, 'I can't help feeling like I would have lost sleep over it.' I also can't help feeling like this would have been an easier explanation if we'd gone somewhere with a sushi train.

'Yeah, you know why? You would have blamed yourself. If don't nobody come to you, what you gonna blame yourself for? If don't nobody come to death row, what are you gonna blame yourself for? You don't know? Come on. What are you gonna blame yourself for?'

'... If nobody comes past and I don't have to do it?'

'Yeah.'

'... Then I haven't done anything.'

'OK. OK, then,' he says, sitting back, looking accomplished, raising his hands like he's resting his case. The bread basket sits between us. 'How can you be accused of something if you did nothing?'

There's a face I do when I've had too much to drink. I squint one eye closed so I can see things in single vision, try to understand the confusing world of a bus timetable or a kebab shop menu. I'm completely sober but I'm doing this face now, trying to pick my way out of a frustrating impasse of questions answered but not really answered. Jerry is chuckling again.

§

In order for his theory to hold that what he was doing was right and good, Jerry had to have complete faith in the justice system. He was not there at the scene of the crime, he was not present in court, he had no place on the jury. He needed to believe that everyone in the chain above him had done their duty and convicted a guilty man in a fair trial. And he did believe the system worked: his faith in it was solidified early, when he was befriended by police officers as a young boy – two black officers who would come to the school to teach judo and karate. They had their own cars – Jerry still remembers their ID numbers: 612 and 613. Nine-year-old Jerry wanted to be a police officer when he grew up, mostly because he wanted to drive his own car. His faith in the justice system was as resolute as his later faith in God.

But two things happened that made him question his belief in judicial accuracy. The first was Earl Washington Jr, a man with the IQ of a ten-year-old, a convicted rapist and murderer, who spent nearly eighteen years on death row before being exonerated by DNA evidence. He was just nine days away from dying in Jerry's death chamber.

Washington Jr's innocence, for Jerry, threw doubt on the others, both past and future. It shook his confidence, but still he did not leave. He had it in his mind that he wanted to get to 100 executions – a nice, round number – before he bowed out. By this point he considered himself an expert and so did others: he was sent to other states, like Florida, to investigate botched executions, correct their method, make sure they weren't using a synthetic sponge. So, he says, given that the first hint didn't work, God threw him a second curveball to tell him he'd done enough: his own trial before a grand jury, a guilty verdict, and fifty-seven months in prison for perjury and money laundering.

Jerry still claims innocence now, in a story that doesn't make sense time-wise or logic-wise, something about a loaded gun hidden in a prison typewriter, peppered as most of his stories are with messages from above. He says his mind was on other things when he was in that witness box: he was mentally preparing to execute ten people in a three-month timespan – the most concentrated number in his tenure as executioner. But he wasn't going to tell the court that. He wasn't going to tell twelve strangers on a jury if he couldn't even tell his wife. There was a storm in his mind when he was being interrogated about a vehicle purchased with drug money he says he didn't know was drug money. But, he thought, if they could convict him of this, they could convict anyone of anything.

That's how his wife eventually found out that her husband had been the state executioner for Virginia for the last seventeen years – a state now second only to Texas in the number of executions carried out since the reinstatement of the death penalty. When his conviction hit the news, she read it in the local newspaper. Jerry still doesn't know who told the press.

§

As the letter to the governor of Arkansas stated, signed at the bottom by Jerry and the many others who worked on death row, the long-term mental-health repercussions for prison staff are not something that tends to be a focus in the death penalty debate. The spotlight generally falls on justice, revenge and the statistically unproven idea of a deterrent. But it's there if you look: short opinion pieces about decades of sleepless nights from former superintendents, the stress and anxiety of practising to kill someone over and over, worrying about it going wrong, living with it going right. Some former executioners become abolitionists, they write memoirs, they travel the world trying to convince those in power to stop the killing. Robert G. Elliott, who executed 387 people while working as a freelance executioner across six states, finished his memoir *Agent of Death* with this line: 'I hope that the day is not far distant when legal slaying, whether by electrocution, hanging, lethal gas, or any other method is outlawed throughout the United States.' His book was published in 1940. Lethal injection was yet to be added to the list.

Prior to the chair and the needle, executions used to take the form of public hangings, but there hasn't been one of those in America since 1936. Many have argued (Norman Mailer and Phil Donahue among them) that if America is serious about killing members of its public, then it should do so with a public audience, perhaps even broadcast the spectacle on television. If we can't see it, we can't truly fathom what is happening, and so it continues to fester below the surface of the judicial system unstopped. Seeing someone die by a planned, bureaucratic method can change minds about the death penalty in a way that hearing about it does not. Albert Camus wrote about the guillotine, about the effect it had on his pro-capital punishment father, who came home from witnessing it in action on a child murderer, vomited beside his bed and was never the same. Camus wrote that if France truly supported the killing of convicted prisoners, it would haul the guillotine in front of a crowd where it used to be, not hide it behind prison walls and euphemistic speech in the breakfast news reports. If France truly stood by what it was doing, he said, it would show its people the executioner's hands.

Jerry spreads his hands now, preacher-like, and tells me that when he left his jail cell four years later, his mind had been changed. 'All of us, everybody in the world, has a death sentence,' he says, calmly. 'Death is promised to all of us. It's guaranteed. It's gonna happen. But the thing is, we don't have to kill to demonstrate to the world that killing is wrong. We know that.' He now believed that not only was the judicial system unfair and flawed, but that the death penalty was, to him, pointless. He offers an alternative punishment: just let them sit in prison, let them suffer for the rest of their lives with the knowledge of what they did. 'On the anniversary date that he took the life of that young lady, that old man, it's gonna come back on him,' Jerry says. 'They gonna live in that cell with him. The walls will start closing in on him. It'll be just like him being in a grave. That's what the guys used to tell me. They said, "Givens, it's just like me getting buried alive." '

Jerry got a new job driving trucks for a company that installs guardrails along interstate highways – another role he sees as saving lives, although this time others would see it that way too. And since his anonymity was blown anyway, he went public with his story. He now travels the world giving talks about the death penalty, about how we don't need it, about what it does to the people who have to carry it out. Morgan Freeman put him in his documentary series about God, in an episode about wrestling with ourselves and our faith in order to do what we believe is right. This week Switzerland wants him, last week it was someone else, today it's me – he's scrolling through his phone showing me how wanted, how needed he is, how he's making good come from the bad because he's someone who's seen it with his own eyes. He still mentors the kids down at his old high school, trying to starve the system of newly condemned. He even wrote a memoir: *Another Day Is Not Promised*. It's filed under 'Religious Fiction'.

Despite all of this, Jerry says he doesn't regret his role in the deaths of sixty-two men – he believes their suffering ended with them. But I suspect it was the beginning of his own. I'm sitting here asking him what it's like, and he can't really talk about it in any meaningful way; he travels the world to talk about it, yet he cannot actually talk about it. Through God, through placing blame on a condemned man's past actions, he has managed to minimise his outsized role as a dealer of death, but there's an enormity here he will not allow himself contact with – he even managed to eat breakfast as usual on execution days. I think he has only half-convinced himself of any of what he's telling me. It's kind of heart-breaking to watch him reason it out over bits of fish and shrimp. What does he do when he wakes in the middle of the night and all he's got is himself?

His specific concern now is the execution team, and when he advocates for the end of the death penalty it is they, the staff, he is fighting for. Jerry is much clearer talking about the pain and torment of colleagues, and sitting there listening to it all, I get the feeling that everything he describes of trauma is also true of him. 'You're holding a lot in, and the average person can't hold that in,' he says. 'A lot of them take their own lives. They turn to alcohol. They turn to drugs. The condemned, he's already gone. You sit on death row for twenty years and psychologically you're already dead – they're ready to accept whatever and get it over with. What you have left is the people that are carrying out the execution. They've got to carry on his death. His death lives through them until they die. It's going to be a part of them, and eventually they will break.'

And break they do. Dow B. Hover, a deputy sheriff, was the last person to serve as executioner in the state of New York. Unlike his predecessor Joseph Francel, whose name was known to the public and who was plagued by death threats throughout his career, Hover's identity remained a secret. He's the one who would change the plates on his car before he left his garage to drive to Sing Sing for an execution. In 1990, he gassed himself in that same garage. John Hulbert, who served as New York's executioner from 1913 to 1926, had a nervous breakdown and retired. Three years later, in his cellar, he shot himself with a .38-calibre revolver. Donald Hocutt, who mixed the chemicals for the gas chamber in Mississippi, was haunted by nightmares in which he repeatedly killed a condemned prisoner while two others waited their turn. He died of heart failure at fifty-five.

'There's nothing like being free from this,' says Jerry. 'If you say it don't affect you, then something is wrong with you. If you don't feel anything from it, then something is wrong with you. The condemned man is gone. He don't have to sweat no more. You've got to sweat, you've gotta breathe, you've got to think about the things that you've been doing.'

We get up to leave, Jerry handing me a box of leftovers and insisting I take them. We follow his slow limp to the door, passing the lobsters, who watch us leave. Clint has been mostly silent throughout dinner – he doesn't usually come with me to interviews, and he didn't want to accidentally derail any of the conversation. But he asks, as I push open the doors to the January cold, if a condemned man can still choose to be killed by firing squad. Sure, says Jerry, but he's not sure where. Maybe Utah.

'But think about it,' Jerry says, standing there in the overlit dark of the car park, holding his own box of shrimp. 'You've got five guys. One live round. But it's gonna be with those five guys for the rest of their lives. They're all gonna think they were the one.'

I slip my gloves on and we wave goodbye. I imagine the full firing squad slipping their gloves on, waving their goodbyes, thinking theirs were the hands of the executioner.

Jerry died of Covid-19 on 13 April 2020. Obituaries link his illness to an outbreak at Cedar Street Baptist Church in Richmond, where he sang in the choir.

The death penalty in Virginia was abolished on 25 March 2021, less than a year after Jerry died.

None of This Is Forever

Death is not a moment but a process. Something fails in the body and the system shuts down as the news spreads – as air is cut off, as blood stops flowing. Decay, likewise, does not happen all at once. No two bodies decompose at exactly the same rate – factors both environmental and personal cause variations across the board: things like room temperature, clothing and body fat all affect the speed of decay. But the basic stages are the same: minutes after death, the cells, now starved of oxygen, begin to self-destruct; the enzymes within turn on the walls that bind them. Three or four hours after death, the drop in body temperature triggers rigor mortis to start its journey downwards, and proteins in the muscles, now without an energy source, lock into place. The eyelids begin to stiffen. Then the face and neck. Twelve hours later the entire body is rigid, spending twenty-four hours, sometimes forty-eight or more, frozen in whatever position it happens to be in. Then, the stiffness vanishes in the order it arrived: eyelids, face, neck. The body relaxes. The next stage – putrefaction – begins.

The embalmer's job is not to halt this process indefinitely but to slow it down. It has been a death practice for millennia all over the planet, with many methods and motives, religious and otherwise. In Europe, bodies were embalmed for reasons of transport, medical science and – in the case of the eccentric eighteenth-century British quack dentist Martin van Butchell – to get around a clause in a marriage contract that said he was only allowed to remain in his wife's property while she was above ground, though this is possibly a rumour of his own making. Either way, in 1775, he had her injected with preservatives and dye, dressed her in her wedding dress and, in his front room, laid her down in a glass-topped coffin with her new glass eyes staring out of it until his second wife, understandably, objected.

Its modern-day popularity in American funerals begins with the Civil War. Until this point in America, much like in Europe, embalming had been mostly used for the preservation of cadavers in medical schools. But as the war escalated and the death toll mounted, bodies of soldiers – both Confederate and Union – overwhelmed hospital burial grounds and were buried by their comrades with makeshift markers, or rolled into trenches near where they fell, theoretically by the victor but then, later, by whoever was nearest: friend, foe, local civilian. Richer families would send for the bodies via the quartermaster general, who would employ a team of men to locate the dead and transport them home; others would travel there to search for the body themselves. At best, they were transported on the railways in airtight metallic coffins or those designed to hold ice, but none of these delayed the onset of decay as much as anyone would have liked on those long trips.

In 1861, when a young colonel called Elmer Ellsworth – formerly employed as a law clerk in President Lincoln's hometown office – was shot and killed as he seized a Confederate flag from the roof of a hotel in Virginia, every aspect of his death was covered by the press, including the unusually 'lifelike' condition of his corpse at the funeral. He had been embalmed by a physician named Thomas Holmes, who had offered his services free of charge. Holmes had spent the years before the war experimenting with a new arterial technique he had learned from a French inventor, Jean-Nicolas Gannal, whose book – detailing his method of preserving bodies for anatomical study – had been translated into English twenty years earlier. Soon after the news about Ellsworth's body got around, other entrepreneurial embalmers set up shop beside battlefields. Holmes himself, who became known as the father of American embalming, claimed to have embalmed 4,000 men for $100 each. In his shopfront in Washington DC, he displayed the body of an unknown man, found on a battlefield, as further advertisement for his services.

When Abraham Lincoln was assassinated in 1865, he too was transported across the country: from Washington DC to his hometown in Illinois, where he was placed in his tomb. It was a three-week trip, passing through seven states and thirteen cities. As he lay in state, his coffin lid open, thousands of people filed past to pay their respects. They could see the work the embalmer had done – this was a dead body, but not as they knew dead bodies to be. Despite the fact that the general mood towards embalmers during the war was one of suspicion and hostility – the US Army received complaints from families saying they had been cheated by embalmers, and at least two were officially charged with the crime of holding embalmed bodies hostage until families paid up – embalming became something aspirational, as well as deeply commercial.

One embalmer in Puerto Rico has since taken it to an extreme, posing bodies like statues at their own wakes: the dead fighter propped in the corner of a boxing ring to show he's still going, the gangster still holding wads of hundreds despite the bullet that killed him. But mostly, the purpose of embalming is to make it look like nothing happened at all. An embalmer's job is to make the dead appear alive but sleeping, to be the art restorer returning the painting to what it might have been – to blur the line between life and death. But if someone is dead, why make believe that they are otherwise?

In 1955 the English anthropologist Geoffrey Gorer wrote in his essay 'The Pornography of Death' that in modern death 'the ugly facts are relentlessly hidden; the art of embalmers is an art of complete denial.' It's been a subject of argument in death writing and embalming textbooks ever since. Later, in 1963, Jessica Mitford published a book called The American Way of Death, which is a very funny but also radical look at the funeral industry, and a pretty ruthless exercise in muckraking. She looked at every part of the industry – anything that could be sold to the consumer for a high price, anything under a baffling name, anything veiled by the illusion that it was a legal requirement and therefore mandatory. She posited that since embalming does not preserve the body indefinitely, and she could not get a straight answer on whether or not an unembalmed body did actually impact the health of the living as many embalmers claimed, embalming merely gave the funeral director something else to sell. The crux of her book was that the funeral industry was preying on the vulnerable.

She may have been opinionated (casually mention her to embalmers and the mood in the room still turns) but she was right about the high cost of death: even now people set up GoFundMe accounts to crowdfund the most basic funerals. If you want, you can sign up for monthly plans to prepay for your own funeral at the cost of a mid-range phone contract. You only need to walk through a Victorian cemetery in London to see how expensive burying someone can get, and how much people were – and still are – willing to pay. Death, of course, can be another way to flaunt your wealth: in Highgate Cemetery, where Nick Reynolds's bronze death masks sit atop headstones, a newspaper magnate lies in a vast mausoleum that deliberately blocks the view from the promenade.

On the subject of embalming, Mitford was wary of funeral directors 'donning the mantle of the psychiatrist when it suits their purposes' in saying that it had a therapeutic effect on the grieving. Reading her book fifteen years ago, I liked her attitude and, having at that point had no personal experience of embalming, I assumed a similar one. It sounded logical to me.

Then, a lovely, retired embalmer called Ron, sitting beside his wife Jean, looked at me across a cafe table and said that he felt hurt when I had described the physical process of embalming as 'violent' in a magazine article. We had been talking for some hours about his life and career, after Dr John Troyer suggested I meet him; Ron Troyer is his father, which has a lot to do with why John is now director of the Centre for Death and Society at the University of Bath. It was his father he spoke about at the dead philosopher's wake, shortly before Poppy told us that the first dead body you see should not be someone you love. John grew up in a house where death was not hidden, and it's very easy to fixate on something that was normal at home but taboo elsewhere – I should know. His parents were visiting from Wisconsin, in February, and were the only people in the crowded Bristol cafe with adequate coats for the light snow outside. Every English person shuffled in looking personally attacked by the weather. I don't pretend to be above this reaction.

Ron is seventy-one, a tall guy with broad shoulders and an expanse of forehead that reminds me of Arnold Schwarzenegger's. Before we got onto the subject of embalming, he had been telling me about the changes in the industry that he had witnessed in the thirty-five years he worked in it. He talked about how the hospice movement in the 1970s – which began in London in the 1960s, with Cicely Saunders, who took it to America – began a shift in our approach to dying, from one of a frenzied medical battle to one of more comfortable acceptance; how when he first started as a funeral director, most deaths occurred in hospitals, with a few on the road or the railway track, but by the time he retired, he was mostly making house calls, calmly sitting with the dying at their deathbeds. He spoke about how the gradual decline in religion over the decades has changed the role of funeral directors, from one of a mere functionary – who dealt with the disposal of the body while the church took care of the soul and grief – to one that now encompasses some kind of bereavement counselling; and how at the University of Minnesota, which he attended himself and where he later taught, the percentage of women in funeral training has gone from almost nothing to 85 per cent of the class.

'When I first started teaching in 1977, if there were women who were coming to the program to learn, they were either the daughter of the funeral home owner or they were married to the son of the funeral home owner,' he says, still ignoring the menu the waiter keeps asking about, because there's a lot to cover in a thirty-five-year career. 'It wasn't that the male funeral home owners wouldn't have hired female funeral directors, but because of the crazy hours you worked, and because of how close you worked, there was a stigma in the industry from spouses about integrating these women. We had to fight that, that was tough. *And* there was the sense that women wouldn't be strong enough physically, or couldn't face it. It was just bull, right from the beginning. Now it's very common to have female funeral directors. It's changed, it's revolutionised.'

'Women brought a lot of compassion that just wasn't there,' adds Jean beside him, who, as a teacher, was not one of the wives who worked in the funeral home, except for two occasions on busy nights when she was roped in to mind the telephones. 'Men are raised to be stoic, but women – it's OK for you to be nice to people because you're a girl.' She rolls her eyes a bit. 'It sounds silly now. But people accepted it more from them.'

Some things never change though: Ron's joked about bribing gravediggers with bourbon to coax them out to work in the frozen Wisconsin winters, and how funeral directors themselves will always be buried in the most expensive caskets available, which they get at wholesale price and rarely manage to sell. 'Finally they get rid of the bronze casket!' he laughed. A lot of Ron's stories are funny but he's also made me cry, talking about working through the AIDS crisis in a small town, watching as families blocked lovers and friends from saying goodbye to the dead. While funeral homes across the country were refusing to take the bodies at all, Ron would stay after hours and sneak in the people who had loved them. 'They were perilous times,' he said, quietly. 'Doing something that might cause community backlash, or take business away from us. We had to be so careful.'

Ron is clearly not a man who values money above all else. He bribed the clergy at Thanksgiving with free turkeys like every funeral director did, but at that time it was the clergy who recommended you to the families of the dead. 'If the clergymen didn't like you, you were outta luck, kid. You were not going to get the funeral.' This is a man who helped bereaved parents dress their dead children, who remembers now, in the cafe, the small, missable detail that when parents of autopsied babies saw the incision on the tiny body, they always referred to it as a 'scar' – implying healing; it was heartbreak in syntax. Outside of the funeral home, he would help support groups for young widows and for parents of murdered children; he was a person who could talk about the darkness when few would. And when a fifteen-year-old girl was killed in a car accident, he went to the school's principal and pleaded with him to allow her class to attend the funeral, explaining the importance of them being there, of seeing, how it was all a part of each student's own grieving process to be present. The family only found out he had done this later; I read it in a thank-you letter he showed me, written by the girl's mother.

Ron didn't see embalming as an act of violence, as I had described it in the magazine article, the one he keeps bringing up to cheekily have a go at me. 'I always thought it was an act of compassion,' he says now. 'I embalmed both of my parents.'

'Was that … therapeutic?' I ask, borrowing a word Mitford had argued about.

'Well, let's see…' he says, pulling an exaggerated thinking face. He smiles. I already know what's coming. 'It wasn't *violent*.'

He said he could not personally show me what the process entailed, as he was long finished in the business, but he urged me to try and find someone who would. I was missing something, he told me, if I was only reading about it.

If anyone was going to convince me that embalming was more than a commercial thing, it would be Ron. But I can't help feeling that hiding the dead body with artifice implicitly agrees with the idea that some truths are too awful to face – and while there are awful truths, I'm not sure that death is one of them. Then Ron told a story about the 'unviewable' body of a Vietnam soldier, one of nine he received that year when he was just twenty-two years old himself. At the father's insistence, he had pried off the bolted-down metal lid of the transport coffin so that the father could see the dog tags and the bag of burned bones and tissue that remained of his son. 'Sometimes what we see isn't what they see,' said Ron. 'What I learned in the work I did was that people are much stronger and much more capable of doing things than we give them credit for.' Ron was not simply telling me that dead bodies should never be seen as they are.

I wondered if there was another thing at play here, that maybe the role of the modern embalmer had been overlooked, regarded as merely mercenary because their work was difficult to see, apart from on a bill. Perhaps there really is a psychological reason for it, I thought, if in embalming both of his parents, Ron was both the family member paying for the funeral and the practitioner of the service.

§

Dr Philip Gore pokes his head out of the door of his office and says he'll be with me in a minute. It's a little before 9 a.m. in Margate, a town on the coast of south-east England with a flat, sandy beach and an iconic amusement park called Dreamland, though it's a little early for sunburned tourists to be crowding the pavements clutching oversized teddy bears and ice cream. It's here that Dr Gore's family have, since 1831, been involved in the funeral industry – first in funereal apparel, then in the embalming and burying of the local dead. He is tall and thin, owlish in his glasses, and I'm early; he won't come out into the quiet of the reception area until his silk vest is buttoned all the way – until his costume, as if he were an actor in the wings, is perfect. It's this theatrical aspect to funerals – the horses, the plumes, the ceremony – that drew him into the family business in the beginning. He says he liked the 'pomp and pageantry' of it all, the presentation of a carefully curated image. He too embalmed his own father.

We settle in his office. As vice president of the British Institute of Embalmers, Dr Gore is also a teacher of embalming's history and, as his PhD in the subject will attest, he is someone who has spent decades thinking about why embalming exists in its current form and what social factors have led to its invisibility. It wasn't always this way: in the 1950s and 1960s – in his father's time – he says that people were more in tune with the reality of nature's course, partly because of the proximity of war, but also because the dead were not taken away by the funeral home. The dead stayed in the community, they stayed in their houses – the coffin placed in the sitting room, ready to receive their final guests. Gore Sr and his team would travel around instead of staying static in their office. 'When things got to the point when it was a bit ... *challenging*, they would screw the coffin lid down,' says Dr Gore. 'Because that was the only option you had. We're in the twenty-first century now. There's a lot you can do to mitigate that.' Forty years ago, in the early days of his own career, he remembers moments when 'the brute reality' of decay made itself known in the form of a puddle at the crematorium, or in the back of a hearse. 'It may have been real, but it wasn't particularly comfortable.' He pulls a face like a judgemental aunt experiencing a sub-par baked good.

Back then, funerals happened within four or five working days, so embalming was less common. Now, somewhere between 50 per cent and 55 per cent of bodies in the UK are embalmed in a typical year (experts estimate it to be similar in America, though the industry doesn't publish statistics) because funerals take longer to arrange, partly due to the paperwork involved in certifying a death, and also because of the difficulty in scheduling. In the quiet area of Thanet, the district that surrounds Margate, there are 110,000 people, sixteen funeral homes (six of which belong to the Gore family) and only one crematorium – organising a funeral in less than three weeks is rare. 'It's very difficult to put the schedules together, unless you want a funeral at half past nine in the morning,' he says. 'Who wants to travel from the back of nowhere to get here for *half past nine*? And refrigeration is a wonderful technique, but I don't know what the contents of your own fridge would be like after three weeks away. You may not want to open the door.' He grins softly and clasps his hands under his chin. I picture Adam in the mortuary, how he had been dead for over two weeks but only smelled of death when we moved him.

Dr Gore speaks with a deliberate delicacy, the product of forty years of practised sensitivity, of figuring out how much the person sitting on the other side of his desk wants to know. The funeral industry is full of euphemistic speech – another thing Jessica Mitford loathed – but he uses none of it on me, and I thank him for it. 'Well, nobody in your family has died today for you to come to see me,' he says, smiling. 'So we're in a different sort of environment.'

He tells me that if I were one of the bereaved, he would describe the process of embalming as something akin to a blood transfusion. People tend not to ask much more after that.

Now, what he calls 'the brute reality' of death is so hidden from us that it's not something we would even worry about confronting at a funeral. In England and Australia, coffins at funerals are usually closed – unlike in America where mourners can pass by the open lid and peer in at the dead, as they did with Abraham Lincoln. Death here is more of a quiet, family moment than a public event. Fewer people will see the body, if any choose to at all. If they do, it will be laid out in the Chapel of Rest, those small rooms in the funeral home (religious only if you want them to be) where visitations take place. It's there they might see the work of the embalmer, not that many would notice it even if they themselves agreed to the 'hygienic treatment', as it tends to be called in the funeral arrangements. The final result is so ordinary, so normal-seeming, that there would be no clue as to the astonishing technical abilities that go into creating that image of normality – or so Dr Gore tells me. I, of course, have no idea what we're actually talking about. I haven't seen an embalmed body to compare to what it looked like in its untouched state. I've seen swollen, embalmed medical cadavers in real life, but that's a different kind of thing altogether – they are preserved for utility, not with the aim of remaining faithful to how they looked to family and friends. I've seen photographs of notable embalmed dead: Lenin's incorrupt-ible body in its glass box – dead for nearly a century, yet largely un-changed thanks to ongoing preservation work. A sleeping Aretha Franklin, her glittering heels raised on a white pillow at the end of her shining gold casket. Rosalia Lombardo, who died of the Spanish Flu one week shy of her second birthday, and was the last body to be shelved away with the monks in the Capuchin catacombs of Palermo, Sicily. She lies in a tiny, glass-topped coffin and has only very recently started to discolour. But what is anyone gaining from seeing a dead body made to look alive?

Dr Gore believes that with the same dwindling religious element in funerals that Ron Troyer observed, the body of the dead has become more significant in the grieving process, and therefore, so has the embalmer. 'In mainstream religious life you've got a two-part individual: you've got the body and you've got the soul. If you don't believe in the soul, all you've got left is the physical individual,' he says. 'And until the funeral, there is still this ongoing sense that they have died but they're still there. There is some sort of relationship continuing for those who need to do that, in the Chapels of Rest.'

Dead bodies are not dangerous, or unhygienic, to be around – despite what many embalmers may have claimed to Jessica Mitford – and Dr Gore isn't suggesting that they are now. There is no legal requirement for a body to be embalmed, unless it's being repatriated overseas and the country receiving the body insists on it. But Dr Gore believes the final image is important. 'If you haven't seen your mother for a long time because you live abroad – which is one of the reasons people take so long to get together – to come and have a few moments with her can be really helpful.'

'And your last picture of her is not—'

'—the desperate image. It is disguising reality, but the irony is, if you said to people, "We're not doing any of that, this is the way she really looks," would that help people? I'm not sure the answer would be yes.'

I think about it for a moment and try to imagine what I would want to see, or what I would expect to see. When I saw the dead bodies at Poppy's mortuary they looked dead, and I didn't find the sight of them, on their own, traumatic – but then again, I didn't know those people in life. I wonder if the process of acceptance in watching someone die over time, becoming gaunt and different, would be undone by seeing them look alive, however briefly, in their coffin. 'I find honesty to be a reassuring thing,' I say. 'Am I alone in this?'

'Completely not. But the issue is that what people assume to be honesty and what is, occasionally, the shocking reality, is quite different,' he says, very patiently. 'There's the irony that we've produced this unknown world. Every dead actor in a film is a live actor pretending to be dead. That is not the way individuals routinely look once they've died. But the public don't know that. Or they've failed to realise that. The embalming process has been in this country for about 150 years; it's a bit late in the day to say, "Let's not do that, we need to get back to our real roots." '

Dr Gore says he'll put me in touch with an embalmer who will show me the process – he tends not to deal directly with the dead so much any more; as captain of this particular ship, his attention is required more in the steering. I thank him and promise that I won't turn it into some horror story, which is something almost everyone I've approached for this book has feared, and which is why I got up before dawn to drive three hours to this seaside town to go through what I suspect is some kind of vetting system. It's taken me five months to speak to an embalmer, but it's understandable: journalists and editors have been sensationalising those who work with the dead for as long as anyone can remember. Even I have, over the years, had to talk editors down from clichéd embellishments of 'hushed tones' and tall, sombre giants who greet you at the creaking door like Lurch, the Addams Family butler. But the British Institute of Embalmers is keen to get the reality of the process not exactly in the public eye, but available to anyone who is interested – their expectations of journalists may be decidedly low, but they want to educate. I'm grateful and apologetic.

'Let's face it,' he says, walking me to the front door. 'We're all producing a manufactured world of some kind. You're producing a word picture. Ours involves the dramaturgy of the funeral.'

§

A month later, I'm waiting out the back of another south London funeral home, by the open roller-door of a garage filled with gleaming black hearses and limousines. A man in a dark suit sits on a fold-out chair, scrolling through his phone, a radio playing at his feet. A young woman with neatly pinned hair, a business skirt and thick beige tights, despite the heatwave, smokes a cigarette over a railing and stares at nothing. Kevin Sinclair emerges smiling from between the bins and smuggles me in through the back door rather than announcing my existence to the front desk. He's in his early fifties, wearing a blue-and-red-check shirt tucked into blue jeans, with glasses and gelled hair. He's been a qualified embalmer for nearly thirty years and a teacher with his own embalming school for half of that, though he seems more like someone you'd split a bag of scampi fries with in the local pub than someone who would show you how to embalm a body.

He leaves me for a moment by the wooden arched door to the Chapel of Rest, next to the staff toilets – one bearing the sign 'DON'T SPRINKLE WHEN YOU TINKLE' and a cartoon bear, winking. A large pine coffin is wheeled past me, disappearing through double doors to be slid back into the refrigerator, where it will stay until the hearse collects it. I can hear two of the funeral home employees arguing with each other in the driveway, some-thing about a family unable to pay for a funeral, something about them being stuck in a hell of probate.

'All he has to do is prove that the family can pay for it.'

'Fuck's *sake*.'

This is the business end, the unquiet voices you only hear out the back, during a break. Inside the office, in the part where the families go, you don't even hear the sound of your own feet on the carpet.

Kevin waves me into the prep room and introduces me to his former student, Sophie, who will be working while we watch. Most of his students these days are women. She's shy and a bit nervous to have me there. She smiles and waves briefly, small col-ourful tattoos flashing between the sleeve of her purple scrubs and the cuff of her nitrile gloves, before turning back to the body laid out between us: the pale, long remains of a man who died of lung cancer three weeks ago. Neat, dark pubic hair fans out across his belly that has, over the last few days, been slowly turning green.

Sophie has spent the morning going through the same process as we did at Poppy's, removing all tubes and hospital ID bracelets. She's also washed and blow-dried his hair, which now looks fluffy and soft. But there is more to do here before the man is dressed. She has already placed some eye caps under his eyelids, the small

convex plastic shields that give the illusion that they have not sunk.
When Mo at Kenyon was explaining why visual identification of
bodies is unreliable, this is the kind of thing he meant: we instinctively look at the eyes of our person, and the eyes of the dead
are not as we remember them. These are not the oysters I saw in
Adam's face when I dressed him for his coffin – these look like
living, sleeping eyes. These are the eyes that Nick the death mask
sculptor hopes to find when he arrives to cast a face. If they're not
here – whether by biology or eye cap – he has to create them.

Now Sophie is tying his jaw together so his mouth doesn't hang
slack. It's a fiddly, invasive procedure to do – one that requires the
embalmer to be face to face with their dead person – and even
more fiddly to describe. She opens the man's mouth as wide as it
will go, his head tipped backwards, and then inserts a large curved
needle with a line of suture thread under his tongue, behind his
bottom teeth, pushing it through the flesh until it exits below his
chin. She then turns the needle around and goes back up through
the same hole, but directs the needle to emerge behind his bottom
lip so the thread is looped around the U-shaped bone at the front
of the jaw. She pulls the string taut so the slack bottom jaw will
be controlled by whatever the thread is anchored to, which, in a
moment, will be the upper jaw. She inserts the needle under the
man's top lip, into the left nostril. She then passes it through the
septum, into the right nostril, and finally it emerges under the top
lip again. She pulls the thread tight, the jaw closes, the ends of the
strings are tied and tucked behind the man's lips. From the outside – unless you knew what you were looking for, directly under
his chin – it looks like nothing has happened at all.

It's not a scary or gross thing to witness, even though the idea
of having my mouth sewn shut, of being made mute, is one
of pure terror; if he were alive during this it would be torture,
there would be muffled screaming. While peering over Sophie's
shoulder, I couldn't help but make strange jaw movements as
I watched, as if proving to myself that I was not the one on the
table. But even though I know this man is dead, and he no longer
has a use for his mouth or his voice, I find it both touching and

sad that he is lying there, limp and unresisting. You could do any-thing to a dead body and all they are doing here is trying to make him look like himself.

Kevin and I are standing on the other side of the room now, out of Sophie's way, leaning against a steel bench piled with papers and plastic tubs of more papers. There are no windows: in this bright white box you are cut off from the external world, vacuum-sealed in your own one. In winter, their busy time, embalmers can be expected to arrive at 4 a.m. and stay until 10 p.m. While their hands are occupied, the only connection to the outside is a radio; they judge the weather from the clothes of the delivery men.

I can't see it yet but I can smell it: embalming fluid, that alien yet familiar smell, the combination of high-school biology labs and a sharp tang of nail varnish that will get stronger as the pro-cedure progresses. When I get home later, I'll notice my jeans stink of it with a strength that invades the whole room. Kevin explains that the formaldehyde gas that evaporates from the fluid is heavier than air (I nod, having learned this from Terry at the Mayo Clinic, as he showed off the floor-level ventilation system in the anatomy lab), but old pre-health and safety embalming rooms placed the air filters high on the walls, assuming all fumes travelled upward, meaning they would only start to filter out long after the gas had filled the room from the ground up and the embalmer's head was in the cloud. Kevin's voice is deep and croaky, a vibration you could hear through walls; this, he says, is the product of decades of chemicals at work on his vocal cords as he worked on what he estimates is over 40,000 bodies. 'I'm actually eighty-four. I'm just very well preserved,' he grins.

'There's three reasons why we embalm,' he says, getting back to the body in front of us, holding up his fingers in teaching mode. 'Sanitation, presentation, preservation. What Sophie's doing at the moment is, she's just setting the features. We want a good facial presentation of what we think the person should look like. Obviously not knowing them, we have to look at the clues in regards to how they hold themselves.' I ask if they ever have photographs to work from. 'Sometimes,' he says. 'Normally it's just guesswork and looking at the deceased. We have photos for things like reconstructions, so we can get measurements and skin tone.' Later he will tell me about piecing a skull together like a jigsaw, wiring the pieces of bone one by one, for a man who played chicken in front of a train, and in front of his two young sons. He says he tries not to judge people on their deaths, but sometimes it can be difficult.

The man is still rigid – the cool of the refrigerator has slowed down decomposition, temporarily extending the state of rigor mortis that would come and go more quickly in the sun. Sophie lifts his long legs into the air one at a time and bends them with force at the knee. It sounds like an old leather wallet being twisted in white-knuckled fists. 'You only have to do it once and then the rigor mortis doesn't return,' explains Kevin. The proteins, once snapped, do not knit themselves back together.

When starting work on a body, the embalmer assesses the situation: how long the person has been dead, how long until their funeral, and whether or not there was any drug intervention – legal or otherwise – that might alter the efficacy of the chemicals in the embalming fluid. They consider the weather both where they are and where the person is going: is it hot and humid? Is it February or July? Are they a holy man who will be taken on a tour of various temples? They do their mental calculations and settle on a concentration of liquid: one that will halt the process of decay so that the person can be transported across the world, or across town, and arrive in the same condition. Too weak and you risk putrefaction, too strong and you risk dehydration – the art is in the balance. The stronger the fluid, the longer the body remains suspended in time, but none of this is forever.

The fluid, depending on what it is, might last longer than the body itself. Those embalmed men returned from the Civil War continue to leach arsenic – a long-ago-outlawed ingredient – into the soil around them, which goes on to contaminate the groundwater. These days in the US, more than 3 million litres of embalming fluid, complete with carcinogenic formaldehyde, are buried every year.

In 2015, flooding in cemeteries in Northern Ireland brought the chemicals to the surface, prompting environmental campaigners to call graveyards 'contaminated spaces'. My gut reaction to view embalming with suspicion is not purely about hiding the true face of death, but wondering whether any of this is worth it.

The Western funeral industry does not have the monopoly on injecting bodies with chemicals to preserve them. Caitlin Doughty, in her book *From Here to Eternity*, wrote about death practices around the world, and there was one place in particular where embalming played a large role. In Tana Toraja, Indonesia, families periodically take the dead out of their tombs to wash and dress them, offer them presents, light their cigarettes. In the period between death and the funeral, a body can be kept at home – sometimes for years. As a trained embalmer and funeral director herself, Doughty was interested in both the emotional element and the practical. She found that these bodies were, in the past, mummified by a technique similar to one taxidermists used to treat animal hide in order to make the skin strong and stiff: oils, tea leaves and tree bark. Now they are mostly embalmed with the same chemicals I can smell in the prep room here in south London. But given that those bodies in Indonesia have a reason to be preserved – that they will be met again by their family, propped up and danced around during a festival – Doughty, echoing Mitford, asked the excellent question: what is the point of preserving a body as intensely as we do here?

This body, lying in front of me, is not being preserved to last centuries in a vast pyramid or to be hauled out of his coffin twenty years from now for a party. He just needs to get through the funeral, which is taking place on the other side of the world. Sophie has selected a fluid on the stronger side to make it happen.

Next she makes two small incisions at the base of the neck to locate the common carotid artery on the right and left: these are the vessels you feel with your fingers when measuring a pulse, and again my hand moves unthinkingly to my neck to feel them. She lifts these blood vessels out of the neck – they look a bit like udon noodles – and slides a thin steel tool underneath to hold them slightly proud of the skin surface, the arteries stretched tight like a rubber band. She ties a thread around each of them so that the fluid can only move in one direction, and inserts clear tubes downwards into the vessels – the head, elevated on a neck rest, will be embalmed separately by reversing the tubing. Using the arterial system as a delivery mechanism, the candy-pink-coloured fluid flushes through the body to replace the blood. The veins, aided by the pressure of the incoming liquid, push the blood towards the unbeating heart, where it pools in its chambers.

'No two deceased will embalm the same,' says Kevin, as the level in the tank slowly lowers. 'Everyone's an individual. Mother Nature's laid out the arterial system slightly differently in everyone. You could have twins and they would embalm totally differently because of the randomness of nature – the general layout of the arterial system could be different, the heart valves could be open or shut at the time of death.' He speaks with the confident certainty of someone who has done this job over 40,000 times. Sometimes the embalming fluid goes through the body in the first attempt, sometimes it doesn't – time makes blood clot and paths close. The same paperwork that delays Dr Gore's funerals means that most embalmings take place weeks after death – again, usually three – unlike in Ireland, where the dead might still be warm, or in America, where Kevin says they consider most of the bodies he works on in England 'unembalmable'. But there are six points of injection around the body – the neck, the upper thigh and the armpit – and a dead end in one direction doesn't mean the journey is over.

While the embalming machine whirs, Sophie massages lanolin lotion into the man's skin – it helps with the dehydration, and the manipulation encourages the embalming fluid to travel through the blood vessels and settle in the muscles. Rubbing his hand, the white of his palm blooms pink. She watches for changes in the skin's colour, or for places where it doesn't, which would indicate a blockage. She massages more lotion into his face and arms, constantly taking a look at the whole picture, like a painter before an easel.

It takes about forty minutes for the fluid to flood through the pipes of his body. Watching it is like a trick of the eye: it happens so imperceptibly that I cannot see it if I don't look away periodically so I can see it afresh. In slow stop-motion, I watch a dead man come back to life, age in reverse: his skin becomes plump, the pink in his veins gives the illusion of warmth, his face is no longer shrunken skin stretched over bony features. 'Shit, he's so young,' I say in shock, then apologise for swearing; maybe it's because I'm new here, but it feels bad to swear around the dead, like I'm swearing in church. No one seems to mind. Kevin reaches over boxes of supplies behind us to grab the death certificate off the top of a stack of papers. What I thought was a frail man in his seventies with oddly dark hair is actually a man in his forties. Cancer had ravaged him, and dehydration had sucked any remaining youth out of his face.

He looks not unlike my boyfriend, Clint, and this situation now feels decidedly stranger. I remind myself that this is not the dead body of someone I love. Months later I take a chance and see if the name I heard in the prep room would bring up an obituary on the internet. There, beside it, is a photo uploaded by someone who did love him. He's tall and fit, smiling. I wondered when his family had last seen him, if they had watched him shrink in life. I cannot imagine knowing the man in the photo and seeing him as he was in the mortuary, when I first met him. He was a different person – a body, destroyed from the inside out. He looks better embalmed, this is undeniable. But I'm still not sure I buy the psychological purpose of injecting chemicals into a dead body for cosmetic purposes: surely seeing the evidence of what he endured at the end of his life is not only part of his story, but part of your process of understanding and grieving?

Out of my head and back in the prep room, Sophie makes a small incision in the abdomen, before picking up a twenty-inch metal rod called a trochar – it has a pointy sharp end, with multiple holes near the tip and transparent tubing that runs from the handle to a machine behind her. She inserts it and guides it blindly, by muscle memory, into the right atrium of his heart. A sucking noise fills the room as a plastic jug in the machine collects a mixture of blood and embalming fluid. 'The more blood we can remove, the better the embalming,' explains Kevin – blood contains bacteria, and bacteria equals decay. The buzzing of the blood aspirator gets louder and Kevin has to shout over it. 'ALTHOUGH YOU'RE NOT GOING TO GET AS MUCH BLOOD AS YOU THINK! BECAUSE HE'S BEEN DEAD SO LONG – BLOOD STARTS TO SEPARATE INTO ITS COMPONENT PARTS!' Sophie pulls the trochar out of the heart and repositions it to pierce the trachea, tipping the man's head backwards to straighten out his windpipe. It releases a sound like a gasp – but this, I'm assured, is from the machine, not the man. She packs the windpipe with a kind of cotton wool, poking it through his nostrils with tweezers, creating a vacuum so nothing will leak. As I watch, my breath catches in my throat imagining the dryness of that cotton. Kevin tells me it's the same stuff as the inside of babies' nappies.

I'm still marvelling at the pink in his fingertips, how soft his once-shrivelled hands look, when Sophie takes the trochar and turns her attention to the abdominal cavity: puncturing internal organs so there won't be a build-up of gas inside them, and sucking out more fluid. This is the bit that looks – you cannot deny it – violent; it looks like stabbing, though Kevin would, in describing it to families, liken it to liposuction. They don't do this in anatomy school embalming – it destroys the organs the students are there to study. She pours the blood down the sink, clots sticking to the bottom of the plastic measuring jug. I notice that there's four litres of it (is it less than I expected? I have no idea) and also that it hasn't made me feel remotely queasy. I'm absolutely fine. I figure it's one of those tricks of the brain where fresh blood from a shallow cut on a live person would make me feel worse than a jug of clotted blood from a dead one in a sterile room. This is blood, obviously, but not as I know it.

Finally, Sophie injects green cavity fluid into the abdomen. It's a more highly concentrated version of the chemicals she's been using so far, and it will firm up the man's belly, making it as solid as the bench that Kevin raps his knuckles on to demonstrate. 'The family will hold his hands, touch his face,' he says. 'Those parts will be softer.' Sophie sutures the incision with medical superglue and looks up shyly, finished. She will do this whole process another six times today.

Over the next twenty-four hours this man will lie in the refrigerator and the colour will even out over his body. He will no longer look like he's just stepped out of an overly hot shower. The tissues will set and plasticise. He will appear alive, only sleeping. And, despite what he's just been through, he'll look more like himself than he did when I arrived.

§

The ubiquitous box of Kleenex sits on the table between us in the family room as Kevin explains how the technology has changed for embalmers over the decades he's been doing this: ventilation of prep rooms is one of them, but there's also the safety of the fluids used, and the hardware. Since it's a process that's almost surgical, as medical implements improve, so too do embalming ones. And more recently, on the cosmetics side, as contestants on TV shows get airbrushed with silicone-based high-definition make-up, so too do the bodies: what stops singers being washed out under bright lights brings skin colour back to the dead. But really, when you strip it back to the essentials, an embalmer can work anywhere. They can embalm in a hut in the jungle with no electricity, using a mobile kit with hand pumps while the rest of the disaster response team drags victims to the shore – in the warehouse at Kenyon, Mo had shown me their kit. They can embalm in the wake of a tsunami, in a hotel room, in a war zone, using the same tables I saw stacked high on those shelves. They can do everything I just witnessed in this funeral home in Croydon in the midst of the most catastrophic events on earth. It's not a huge production. It's just them and a corpse.

In a mesh tent on a faraway island Kevin has embalmed the drowned passengers of a plane that crashed into the sea, people who would have survived if they had not inflated their life jackets inside the plane and become trapped within it, glued to the ceiling as the ocean rushed in. He's peeled the shirt off a man who knew a flight was going down but had the foresight and the steady hand to write a letter to his wife on the fabric, knowing that a piece of paper would disintegrate or be lost, but a shirt had a chance of being recovered with him. He's looked after the bodies of British soldiers in Afghanistan, realigning broken bones and charred pieces, reconstructing full limbs inside a uniform to send them back to their mothers.

'It's the last thing you're able to do for them,' says Kevin. 'Give them some dignity. It's a privilege to do things like that. What we do, to the outside world, looks very aggressive. But part of the grieving process is recognition. We want the deceased to be looking their best for the family, so they can move on. They've had the disbelief, and the anger, and the tears. It's helping them in their journey.'

I ask him the same thing I asked Dr Gore, if it might be harmful for someone to see the dead body looking dead. He says some-times it can be a shock that doesn't help. People don't want to think about the car crash, or the suicide, or the cancer; they want to think about the life before that – the football match, the after-noon tea. Kevin says his job is to trigger memories so that the focus is on loss, rather than the manner of death.

'What we want to do is impact their senses, so as well as how they look is how they smell: aftershaves, perfumes,' he says. 'Maybe someone wears a specific scent, and even before you see them you know they're in the vicinity because you can smell them. It's all triggering memories.' It's true that scents can make you time-travel – I have walked past men in the street who smell of turpentine, and suddenly I am at my father's feet, thirty years ago, watching him paint with cheap oils that he later complained never dried.

Memories also hide in the folds of clothes. Kevin has embalmed and dressed a Father Christmas. He has gently eased the body of a very elderly lady back into the dress she was married in: sewn by her own hand from the silk of abandoned German parachutes, saved up for when her man came back from the war.

In America, cosmetics are a major operation in the embalming process – I saw an advert in the back of one of the magazines at Kenyon for a paint colour palette that 'visually elevates sunken eyes' and thought briefly about buying it, before I remembered what I was looking at – but traditionally it is less so in the UK. If someone wants it done, Kevin asks them to bring in the dead person's make-up, and then he plays detective in the prep room. 'We won't actually ask any questions, but we'll open it up and look at it. There'll be four or five lipsticks and one that's just a nub. That's your favourite one. There'll be an eyebrow pencil about that big –' he pinches his fingers together and squints like he's crushing an ant – 'that's their favourite. Eye shadow, you've got several shades, but there'll be one that will be worn down to the silver. That's the one.'

There's a pause. I can't help it, I have to say it. 'I think you're a brave man drawing a woman's eyebrows on.'

He shakes his head, laughing at the absurdity of eyebrows. 'It's so hard! Why do you pluck them out and put them back on again? I don't understand.' I assure him that some of us learned our lesson in the early 2000s.

I think back to Ron Troyer and Phil Gore embalming their own parents, how two people who are aware of the artifice of embalming still went through the process with their own dead. Neither said they did anything differently. But I wonder, now, if it is technically more difficult to embalm someone you know, when you knew their face so intimately in life.

'It is harder when you know someone,' says Kevin. 'Not because of the process but because you could picture them as they were, and they never look the same. I do a lot of celebrities for one company I work with, and I get mega-critical of what I do because I've got a picture of how they were on stage. They look different because the muscle tone is gone, they're holding themselves differently. I stay longer to achieve that picture in my head. I'm never happy.'

I ask if he ever thinks about his own death, and he gives me a joke answer about his funeral plans: a coffin with each side bearing a multi-angled life-size photograph of him naked but for his Y-fronts. 'I just want to make people laugh. I've seen too much sadness,' he says. I try again and ask him if he thinks about dying. He says not really, but if someone he knows announces a cancer diagnosis he extrapolates the graph to its worst-case scenario, because that is all he sees. You don't get a cancer survival story in the prep room: you just see, as Kevin calls it, 'the inevitable end point'.

The dead have surrounded Kevin all his life. His parents ran a funeral home, and the family lived in the flat above. He remembers being sent downstairs on a Sunday, the day when the flat was cleaned, to fetch the hoover from a cupboard under the stairs. He'd have to walk right past the dead people, laid out in their coffins in the Chapel of Rest. He doesn't remember ever being scared of the bodies, but he knew instinctively not to talk about it outside the house. 'Kids just didn't understand what my parents did, so it was up for ridicule,' he says. Even now he doesn't talk about what he does – he's only talking to me because I asked him to, or rather Dr Gore did – and instead of 'embalmer' he says he's a teacher, if anyone asks. 'There's a denial of death in England,' he says. 'They don't want to know us unless something happens, then we're their best friend for the next two weeks. After that, we don't exist again.'

He didn't immediately follow his parents into funeral service, but he was never really apart from it. When he was tall enough to carry a coffin, he'd earn £15 as a freelance pallbearer and spend it all on records at HMV. When he left school, he became a stone-mason, carving angels into the headstones that will stand in cemeteries for longer than any of us will live. He made the monument you look at, the place you return to, the thing you address your monologue to in the cemetery when your person is under the ground. Now his work is something you see for a minute, then it's gone.

'As an artistic person, don't you feel sad that your best work gets buried or burned?'

'No,' he says abruptly. 'Because I've already...'

He pauses, thinks about it a bit longer.

'Here's one that happened a few years ago,' he says. A man had been in an industrial accident, his head and torso crushed while attempting to free a jam. His wife had to identify him as he was, after he had been pulled from the machine. 'It was … just a mess. She said to me, "Is there anything you can do?" I told her I'd do the best I could.'

Later, he received a letter.

'Thank you. It wasn't perfect. But you gave him back to me.'

Love and Terror

In the Egyptian mummification process, all organs were removed and placed in jars, bar the heart. The heart – considered to be the centre of the person's self, their whole being, their intelligence, their soul – was left in place to be judged by the gods. In the underworld, it was weighed against a feather to see if the person had lived a virtuous life. If it did not make the scales tip, the person was granted entry to the afterlife. If the heart proved heavier than the feather, the goddess Ammit – part lion, part hippopotamus, with the head and teeth of a crocodile – would eat it.

In the mortuary, on the lower ground floor of St Thomas' Hospital, on the South Bank of the Thames, a heart is placed on scales and the result shouted across the room to be recorded on a whiteboard in fading pen. Its weight is determined to be healthy or unhealthy – here you are judged only on what is known and seen by naked eye or microscope. It is not for these people to rule on how you lived, but how you died, on the balance of probability.

This is where the dead body tells its story to someone who is listening: be it murder, suicide, heart attack. It is in places like this that Mo, when he was a detective, would hear that story translated from mute flesh to something he could work with, some evidence to help solve a crime. The manner of someone's death might remain a mystery to most of the death workers I have already met, but here it's their job to find out.

If you die on a level above, the porter transfers you on an inconspicuous sheet-covered trolley to a fridge below. If you die in certain boroughs near the hospital, the ambulance that collects you from the floor, or the bed, or the road, will transport you here. If the coroner requires one, an autopsy or post-mortem examination (they both mean the same thing, one's just in Greek, the other in Latin) will be carried out, in this room, to officially determine how you met your end. If your doctor had seen you shortly before your death and was certain they knew how you died, the death certificate can be completed without taking your body apart. Some bodies are here, untouched by scalpel, waiting for the funeral homes to collect them. Some bodies are unidentified, waiting for a name.

More numbers are being listed aloud in the background, the final results of a woman's lifetime of growing, shrinking, existing. The liver. The kidneys. The brain. The pathologist is slicing samples of organs under a white spotlight and making notes on her clipboard. I'm peering into the empty abdominal cavity of a large man suspected of dying of a stroke. His internal contents lie in an orange biohazard bag between his feet for the pathologist to weigh and inspect next.

When a heart stops beating, blood ceases to flow around the body at the speed of life, but it still moves. Gravity draws it to the bottom reaches – the back, if the person died on it – and there it collects, slowly turning the skin dark like a bruise. When space is created by removing the organs, blood seeps from severed vessels in the arms and legs to fill it. In the recesses beside his spine, where his lungs were, where his kidneys used to be, blood pools thickly. Lara-Rose Iredale helps it along, gently milking his femoral artery for a sample to send to toxicology. Massaging his thigh, she looks like a physiotherapist on the sidelines of a football pitch.

I knew Lara would be the one to show me what they do here. I've known her for years, first as a familiar face with faultless eyebrows who always appeared at death-related talks around the UK, someone who could be counted on to hang around a pathology museum if there was something happening, even if it was just free wine. I became curious about her job at a funeral industry awards ceremony I was writing about, where Lara was nominated for APT (anatomical pathology technologist) of the Year. Her friend Lucy was sitting beside me, and mentioned how much Lara keeps quiet. She told me that Lara had worked on the victims of the 2017 London Bridge attack – where a van deliberately ploughed into pedestrians before the three perpetrators ran through the area around Borough Market, stabbing diners, bystanders and police with twelve-inch kitchen knives – but she never talked about it. Others might talk about their work for internet numbers, broadcast it on social media along with pictures of themselves in scrubs brandishing stainless-steel tools. Lara's Instagram was full of night-out selfies, pictures of her hanging upside down on an aerial hoop, and sometimes a rare glimpse of the huge easy smile that I've come to know her by. She has a tarot card tattooed on each thigh – DEATH and JUDGEMENT – and around Halloween she will draw a little bat in liquid eyeliner on her cheekbone. As for the job, it rarely gets mentioned, though she is clearly in love with what she does. 'Corpse servant' is how she describes it, there in the short bio beside her perfectly painted face. I wanted to know what, exactly, that entails.

The job of an APT is to do the physical work of taking a body apart to assist the pathologist in their investigation: they eviscerate and reconstruct the patient, then clean the body and all of the equipment used in its deconstruction. They are the people you meet if you go to a mortuary to identify a body, they deal with the family and the funeral homes, and they wrestle with the mountain of paperwork that comes with every death and the movement of bodies from place to place. The UK, as everyone keeps telling me, is a paperwork-heavy place to die. Lara says she has nightmares where the dead sit up on their steel trays and try to leave the mortuary; she wakes in a sweat not with the horror of the living dead, but with the paperwork it would necessitate if the bodies went missing.

She began her training here in 2014, shadowing an existing APT, and qualified three years later, learning on the job, leaning over the dead. Trainee placements are rare and hard to come by, and for Lara it took years of waiting and hoping. Now, on top of the regular day-to-day admin work and autopsies, she mentors and teaches the new trainees, walking them through the human anatomy and how it fits together, how it looks when it goes wrong, and what it might mean. Trainee APTs are not the only ones looking over her shoulder – trainee doctors are too. As Terry explained at the Mayo Clinic, the role of the medical cadaver is to give the student a map of a body in working order. Here, they can see what an abnormality looks like, and Lara can show them the reality of a diagnosis: what telling someone they have cancer actually means, what cirrhosis of the liver looks like, what obesity means for your cramped organs, and the shocking visual fact that ribcages stay the same size no matter how big you get. Today she's showing me.

I've been here a while. Earlier that morning, I watched as Lara manoeuvred the hydraulic lift to extract three bodies from the fridge and position them by the sinks that stand in a row in the centre of the room. Even though the mechanical lift moves the trays up and down, there is still physical work in pulling the trays out of the cold with enough strength to get them to slide out. She says the first thing to go in this job is your back: you're not only pulling, you're *leaning* and pulling, and you're pulling not entirely predictable shapes that are unevenly weighted. The mortuary staff have their own health-and-safety training: nobody else in the hospital has to move like these women move. And it is all women here – at least all of the APTs – and they are each, bar Tina the locum who has been in this role for thirty years, covered in tattoos from the neck down, with buzz cuts and piercings and multicoloured hair. They're all young. They all have tickets to the same Rammstein gig.

After the bodies were all in their places, the three APTs began their visual assessments of their designated corpse, which is a constant part of an autopsy: each step of the way they will stop and look for signs of things gone wrong. As the pathologist circled the man, pausing to make notes on a clipboard, Lara searched him for scars, looking for clues of prior surgery or injury that might have something to do with his death. Even nicotine stains on fingers give clues as to how someone might have died. She rolled him in a routine check to make sure there wasn't a knife in his back ('So far we haven't found one, but you never know') and stuck a needle into both of his eyes to take a sample of his intraocular fluid – this, along with the blood and urine, will be sent for testing. Then she sliced him in a Y-shape, starting about two inches below the collar bone, continuing down past the navel, but avoiding the actual navel because, she says, it only causes problems later when she has to stitch him up. She peeled back the skin and, pinching it between her fingers, sliced the abdominal muscle carefully so as not to damage any vital organs beneath it. Using a scissor-like tool – rib shears, like I had seen at the Mayo Clinic – she clamped through the cartilage that separates the breastbone from the rib cage, and lifted it off like a shield to reveal pink, glistening lungs.

I don't know it yet, but from this day onwards I will stop eating ribs – unlike Lara's manager, who I saw happily eating a barbecue rack in the staff room just across the hall. It was not just the visual that got me, but also the sound. If you've ever watched a *Rocky* movie you've heard the rib shears cracking the rib plate, cutting through the cartilage: it is the snapping noise that follows a blow to the chest. A week from now I'll see *Creed II* and the sound that accompanies a slow-motion punch to Donnie Creed's ribs is almost exactly this sound that I heard in the post-mortem room. I'll spend the next twenty minutes of the movie wondering if they took a mic to the morgue.

Next, she tied a string at the duodenum – the beginning of the small intestine – sliced through it on the lower side of the knot, then lifted the bowel out of his abdomen, pulling out all twenty feet of intestines hand over hand like a sailor with a rope. She dropped all of it into the orange biohazard bag. 'Through there is the heart,' she said, pointing with a gloved finger before she leaned over his chest to begin freeing up the structures of the neck.

It takes about an hour to do a standard autopsy – longer for someone who has been in intensive care for a long time, full of tubes and lines whose placements need to be checked too. It's quicker to autopsy a thin person rather than a fat person, simply because their organs are easier to find. But there are some parts that are difficult whatever the body, processes that need both skill and practice. Lara tied off the base of the oesophagus and then used a blunt tool to sever the connecting tissue around the organ, and then further up, separating the neck skin from the muscle. She put the tool aside then slid her hand up under the skin, her every knuckle visible as she worked to find a pocket at the back of the tongue. 'There's no tool that would make this easier,' she assured me, her arm halfway up the guy's neck like a puppeteer, her gaze somewhere off in the corner of the room as she navigated by feel alone in that slimy dark. 'Got it.' She pulled out the tongue using the pocket as a hook, and the tongue and oesophagus, with vocal cords, came out in one piece. It looked like a long fillet of pork. She pointed to a horseshoe-shaped cartilage construction that sits in the throat. Part of an autopsy is to check if this structure is broken: if it is, that would suggest a strangulation. My gloved hand went to my own throat to see if I could feel it bend.

Next she sliced through the diaphragm, and lifted the heart and lungs off the spine in one connected block. Then the stomach – with oesophagus and tongue still attached – liver, gallbladder, spleen and pancreas in another block. These organs joined the others, squelchily, in the bag at their owner's feet. Then, finally, the kidneys, adrenals, bladder and prostate, all connected, all in the bag too.

The smell of a fresh abdominal cavity opened to the world for the first time is hard to forget in the days after you encounter it: it smells of refrigerated meat, human shit and the blended penny tang of blood. Add that to the smell of unwashed skin, groin and open dry mouths that house rotting, unbrushed teeth and you have a whole human body at our base level. Seeing it all come out like this, it's hard to believe all of this stuff makes a person live, and that it can exist without going fatally wrong for so many years. I stare in at the empty space, while the woman on the table beside us has her organs weighed and recorded on the whiteboard. Our guy will be next.

'I look at all of this and wonder how it doesn't just fall out of me,' says Lara, pausing the thigh massage for a moment and gesturing at the bag of organs. She scoops the loose pieces of shit from around the rectum, inside the cavity, and places them on the table next to his leg to deal with later. One nugget falls off the edge and sits precariously close to my boot for the next three hours, until it is washed away with a jet hose, just like everything else. At one point Lara is talking and gesticulating and a sliver of visceral fat flies off her glove and lands on the floor too. This is clearly not a glamorous job, though she discovered it on television: she wanted to be Dana Scully in The X-Files, specifically Scully in the episode 'Bad Blood' where she plays a forensic pathologist, autopsying victims of a drugged pizza murder. 'It's one of the funny ones,' says Lara, who grew up watching late-night TV in the nineties just like I did, and abandoned the idea of becoming a forensic patholo-gist when she learned you had to become a doctor first. Then, even in full-time training, it takes five and a half years to qualify. She wanted to go straight to the mortuary and skip the living entirely.

The man has a history of epilepsy, so Lara figured he was 'a probable neuro case' and said if there was anything to find, it would likely be in his head. 'In the UK you either die in your head or in your heart,' she says, combing a neat horizontal parting in his hair in a line from ear to ear to clear a path for a scalpel blade. She slices the skin, then folds the face down towards his chin, but it seems harder to do than she was expecting, the skin less easy to separate from the bone than usual. Then she uses a circular bone saw and finds that the skull is thicker too. The pathologist comes over and points at the man's folded face, at his dark strawberry birthmark. She says that a birthmark like this happens when the foetus is being formed, when there is little to separate the face and the brain: whatever happens without will be seen within, and in this case everything is slightly fused, the imprint of the birthmark runs through the layers of flesh and bone like a stick of rock. When Lara removes the top of the skull and peels back the thick mem-brane that protects the brain (it's called dura mater, meaning 'tough mother'), there is a dark mark where the birthmark touched. She takes a photo for the pathologist's records and pulls the brain out of the skull. She asks me if I would like to hold it.

I cup my hands together and feel the weight of it. This is the thing that made him who he was, and inside it was the clot that probably killed him. It is flesh-coloured and white, shot through with wormy lines of red and black – this is not the pink of cartoon brains, or the grey matter of high-school biology books, or even the brains in jars in the pathology museum, which are bleached, set, stiff. In my hands the lobes flatten and relax, taking up more space than the dome of the skull would allow. Later, Lara will pack his skull cavity with cotton wool because the brain would never reform the neat shape it once held inside it, a tight case to keep the brain compact and safe. The weight in my hands is cold and heavy, dense but fragile – it moves like jelly. I wouldn't want to press it even lightly for fear of damaging it, yet I've sat through boxing matches and watched blunt impacts to the head knock fighters to the floor unconscious. I think of the wives who insisted their American footballer husbands were never the same after the years of charging head first into other players, how they became violent and confused and nobody saw it but the women. Hold a brain in your hand and you realise how much danger we put them in to score points while others watch and eat hot dogs. I imagine what a bullet would do. I remember Neal Smither, the crime scene cleaner, washing the brain off the side of his grandparents' house, how it hardens to cement and becomes impossible to clean.

I slide the brain off my gloves into Lara's blue plastic bowl. She threads twine under the basilar artery, which protrudes enough to act as a shallow loop, and dips the organ upside down into a bucket, tying the ends of the twine around the handles to suspend it in formalin. Over the next two weeks, it will firm up enough for the pathologist to slice it open – to 'breadloaf' it, like Terry – in search of the cause of death. 'RTB' (return to body) is already written on the side of the red-and-white bucket, and Lara places it on a shelf where it disappears in a crowd of more brain buckets. Everything you came here with leaves with you – organs are put back in the orange biohazard bag after the pathologist has weighed them and searched them for tumours and other malfunctions. And after the abdominal cavity fluids are ladled out like soup from a pot, the bag is placed in the empty space the organs once filled, with cotton wool tucked into the gaps around it. The front of the rib cage is slotted back into place, and the skin sewn up. Weeks from now, when the pathologist is finished with the brain, an APT will undo enough stitches to be able to slide it into the orange bag with the rest of him, and his body will be ready for collection by the funeral home.

Months prior to this I sat at a picnic table in winter as Anil Seth, a neuroscientist, explained consciousness to me. He told me that reality is the brain's best guess at what is happening out-side of its own dark room, where it sits windowless and blind, being fed information by other tools – eyes, ears, fingers. All of your senses are spies for your brain. It pieces together what it can from the scant information it is supplied, blurs it with memory and experience and calls it life. Now, all of this magic, all of this brain's best guesses in the dark, are inaccessible. They are pure organic matter in a bucket, firming up so that someone can slice its billions of forged connections that create reality and wisdom, an entire universe of someone, and find the reason why it all stopped.

On the other side of the room, a tiny organ is being held aloft, pinched between tweezers. A pathologist and two policewomen are judging the weight of a baby's heart.

§

The day before I came to watch Lara work, she emailed me the standard document that she has to send to everybody coming to view an autopsy. It was a warning, along with the suggestion to have a good breakfast and wear thick socks for the wellies. She said she knew that I had seen death before, but even so, I needed to know that this was a specialist paediatric pathology department as well as a straightforward hospital mortuary. Babies and children were sent here from all over, and their post-mortems were carried out in the same room as the adults. It was possible, though she didn't know the schedule yet, that I would see dead children. I said this was fine, I'd seen dead bodies before. I'd seen, at this point, hundreds of them, whole and in pieces.

I was, in hindsight, somewhat cocky.

After she stitched up the man, methodically and neatly, Lara shampooed his hair (Alberto Balsam in sweet strawberry, which from my experience is every mortuary's shampoo of choice – a surreal smell to mix with the abdominal cavity and the formalin of the brain buckets), sprayed him with antibacterial solution and hosed him down. She sponged him, lifting his arms and legs, trying to clean as much of him as possible. She explained that not all mortuaries did this, but here they considered it the right – the *nice* – thing to do. 'You've just had your insides on your outsides,' she says, matter-of-factly, adding that because de-composition is a bacterial process, they figure anything to help stall it is a good thing for the funeral homes and families (not everyone thinks of the chain of death workers like Lara does – embalmers, like Kevin and Sophie, frequently have to hide the effects of careless autopsies or storage). There was antibacterial spray bouncing off his body, a jet of water ricocheting loudly off steel, and I was getting in the way so I backed away from the table. I backed away so far that I found myself beside a baby. He was two weeks old.

I had been watching this baby for the past two hours out of the corner of my eye, trying to keep focused on what Lara was doing as she looked for a pocket inside the neck, as she tied off organs and photographed the brain. The room was large, but not huge; Lara and I were maybe ten feet away. The whole time, I could see it. I could see that a baby's skull does not need to be sawn open like an adult's – nothing is fused, so the pathologist trimmed the thin connecting fibres with scissors and peeled open the five planes of the skull like petals on a flower. Using only his thumb, he levered them up from the fontanelle, that forbidden soft spot on the baby's head that I, age four, remember promising not to touch as I was handed my new sister to hold. I heard one of the police officers say the mother has a history of psychosis, and realised they were looking for evidence that she had killed him. I watched the pathologist fan out the ribcage like a palm frond, separating each rib, sliding his finger along the curve, checking every tiny bone for fractures. I watched as this baby was comprehensively taken apart, his back resting on a block so that his open chest was pushed forward and his open skull thrown backwards while they discussed the findings above him. I could not read the police officers' faces as they perched politely on stools, occasionally making notes, frequently leaving the room.

Now I'm next to him, and a young, green-haired APT is having a hard time putting him back together. She has stitched up his body, but she's having trouble with his face. During the post-mortem investigation, he was cut under the neck in such a way that it changed the way the face now rests on the skull: the bottom lip hangs loose from the chin and the weight of the droop causes one eye to keep opening. The APT has to make him look normal again, pressured by the knowledge that the parents will notice any change, that bereaved parents, in their final visit, try to mentally record every detail they can before the baby is taken away. She keeps closing the eye, pushing at the small pink lip, sighing, trying to get the expression right – the blank serenity of a sleeping baby – and it keeps falling off the bone. Lara pauses her cleaning to come over, and with her calm, patient direction combined with a tube of Fixodent, the younger APT manages it. It shouldn't matter, but the baby is unusually beautiful. I am utterly transfixed by his glued-together face.

As with the adults the babies are washed, not by hose, but in a small blue plastic tub in the sink, as natural as my mother bathing my pink siblings in the kitchen. He sits propped up in the corner, the bubbles almost at his shoulders. The APT leaves him there briefly to fetch something off a shelf and I am left watching as he starts to sink, slowly, his face slipping below the suds. I'm supposed to be observing, not touching – especially away from Lara, in a part of the room where I was not invited nor expected to be – and I stand frozen, unsure of what to do. I try to suppress every in-built urge to stop him drowning, telling myself he is dead, *realising* that he is dead, that nothing I do here would matter or change the outcome of his being dead. He slips below the waterline as I stand stiff and useless, coming undone.

The APT returns, lifts him out of the bubbles and dries him. She lays him on a towel as she collects the things she will need for the next part of the process: a nappy, booties, a romper suit. After dressing him, she slides three plastic hospital armbands over the chub of his hand, holding his tiny fingers as she pushes them further up his limb. She's as gentle with him as you would be with a living baby, supporting his head as normal where babies this age are unable to, but even more so: the pathologist has severed the vertebrae in his neck.

With babies, they usually do put the brain back into the skull – since it has not yet hardened and fused, the space is more forgiving than an adult's. But mostly it's because the weight of a baby's head is something that comes biologically programmed in a human's mind: parents, cradling their child in the viewing room, will notice if the weight of the head is too light. But in this baby's case, a forensic one, the brain needs to be kept for further tests. Lara suspends it in a bucket, just like she did with the adult brain, small and lost-looking, a planet in deep space. Meanwhile, a knitted bonnet is selected from the huge clear Tupperware box of baby bonnets in the corner – lemon yellow, pink, blue, there are hundreds of them – and pushed down over his head to cover the incision that runs across his scalp from ear to ear. I help the APT steady his tiny body, his loose neck.

I thought that the head, now empty, would be relatively weightless – from where I stood hours ago, the bones of the skull were so thin in the fluorescent light as to be almost translucent. But it was not. There was still the soft flesh of his face, the plump rounded cheeks. A baby's head, without the brain, feels sickeningly light and unfathomably heavy.

§

I never found out if the mother did kill her baby, if whatever mental-health issue she had had pushed her to shake him. I do know that his only possession in the world was her breastmilk in a half-filled tiny bottle that was tucked beside him in his card-board coffin, before he was placed back in the designated baby fridge with his name on the door shortly before I left. I peeled off my gloves, waterproof apron, scrubs and wellies, handed back my visor, and Lara congratulated me on not having to step outside at any point. I could stand it. I withstood it. I didn't tell her that all I could smell was the cold meat and shit of abdominal cavity and all I could think about was the baby.

I reverse our steps that morning, back through the green lino-leum corridors, back past a decommissioned gurney with a note on it, up the stairs, through the door and crowd of families waiting, pushing prams, eating packaged sandwiches while they wait in the hospital reception area. I step into the light outside and I feel like I'm under water. Big Ben is visible from the door of the hospital through the thick autumn mist. It stands on the other side of the Thames, wrapped in scaffolding, silenced for the handful of years it will take to restore. This particular bell tolls for no one, cur-rently, but the dead still grow in number every day. Some of them are here.

It seems obvious now, but I had no idea so many of them are babies. I didn't know the infant mortality rate in the UK is, while falling, still higher than other comparable countries. I didn't know that an English soap star campaigned for foetuses born dead before a certain age to have birth certificates as well as death certificates – something that proved they existed, if the parents wanted one. I didn't know that when a baby dies of SIDS (Sudden Infant Death Syndrome), that cause is only ruled because it has been autopsied and every other possibility eliminated. I never really thought about dead babies, or the mothers who lose theirs repeatedly; when I read about miscarriages I thought only about blood and clots, not recognisable organisms with limbs and eyes and fingernails that go to the mortuary and have a designated refrigerator. Lara tells me that she sees some mothers' names turn up multiple times – an-other attempt, another death, another storm in the mother's heart that she will keep quiet because it's not something people talk about, because we don't know how to, because most people are, like me, blind to the reality. I didn't know that small foetuses can be taken apart to find out if there is something, anything, they can do for the mother's future pregnancies so that they will not end like this one. The hope that maybe the problem is genetic, maybe it is preventable, maybe this occurred for some diagnosable reason. Of course all of this happens. *Of course it does.*

I take the train home and stare at the empty seat across from me, avoiding looking at the toddler in the pram by the door and the pregnant woman pushing it. To get deliberately pregnant feels like the most hopeful, reckless thing you can do to your heart. Parenthood, from what I can see, must be a mess of love and terror. The thought of it makes me woozy.

I ask Clint to come over because I need to be reminded that bodies are warm. I tell him about the baby, and about the others – a line of small white cardboard boxes with paperwork resting on top, ready for post-mortems in the afternoon. I tell him about the foetus that was so small that he was resting on a kitchen sponge with his legs dangling over the edge. He was purple, translucent, wet-looking – a half-formed alien face. In the supermarket, buying dinner I won't eat, I burst into tears at the sight of a tube of Fixodent. That night I dream about dead babies wrapped in their blankets, lying in rows on the gravel outside my bedroom window. In the morning Clint tells me I mumbled into my pillow, 'I need to remember they're not real.' Something in my subconscious was in self-preservation mode, rationally dismissing my nightmares, but I woke to remember some nightmares *are* real. I had seen them.

I stay in bed for about three weeks, crawling out only when work forces me to. I try to process why I am reacting like this to something so clearly part of life, of *so many* lives that aren't mine. I don't have any children, and until I saw that baby in the blue tub I didn't feel any desire to. I had never felt any maternal urge until I saw a dead baby, sinking. Waves of thought and possibility crashed in my head and heart as I stood there that day, watching him slip under. I felt seasick.

I needed to figure out why the baby in the bathtub affected me on an emotional level that watching him being autopsied did not.

I told friends about it – in vaguer terms, so as not to transfer the image like a virus – and they said, 'Of course you're upset, you saw a *dead baby*.' But I wasn't upset when he was being taken apart by the pathologist – an objectively more horrific scene. I've seen a headless man, I've seen heads without bodies, hands without arms. I had just held a brain. The emotional reaction I had when I was dressing the dead man for his coffin made total sense to me, and the honour of being there felt like a conclusion to a lot of my thinking. It was confirmation that this was the right thing to do by someone you love, and also a good way of teaching yourself that the dead body is not a thing to be feared. Why is a baby in a bubble bath the thing that knocked me down? I felt like I was being ab-surd. I stopped trying to explain it, I was only making other people feel ill.

In 1980, Julia Kristeva, the Bulgarian-French philosopher, published *Powers of Horror: An Essay on Abjection*, about how a threatened breakdown in order causes a loss of distinction between subject and object, between the self and the other. Something is not where it should be, and the terms of our corporeal reality shift; we be-come horrified. She writes that 'the corpse, seen without God and outside of science, is the utmost of abjection. It is death infecting life.' When the baby was in pieces, to me he was pure biology, pure science, the pathologist was doing his job and everything was in order within the context of that room. But when he was in the tub he was just a baby – it was a life scene, infected by death. The tectonic plates of my reality moved as I stood there. Kristeva had a similar experience visiting the museum that was once Auschwitz. We are all taught what happened there, we are given the sky-high numbers of death and injustice, but the enormity is hard to grasp until you are given something small and familiar, like a pile of children's shoes.

Life is not supposed to surface in the mortuary. Everyone has their bound-aries: some APTs won't read the suicide note in the coroner's re-port, but *all* of the APTs hate it when the bodies are warm, when the patients have been transported from a hospital bed upstairs to the mortuary below and have not spent enough time in the refrigerator to cool their organs. It's physically uncomfortable for them to work on the cold bodies – they each keep a bowl of warm water in the sink, to periodically de-ice their hands – but they prefer it, emotionally. 'Wouldn't it be nicer and easier if they were less cold inside?' I had asked, as Lara stood there, soaking her frozen fingers. She looked visibly repulsed at the thought. 'Nope. Dead bodies cold. Live bodies warm.' Aaron had told me the same thing in the mortuary with Adam. There is comfort in their discomfort – it is what solidifies the distinction between the living and the dead.

To me, the most affecting horror is not the blood-soaked madman with the chainsaw, but the quiet domestic scene gone wrong, the minor note on the piano keys: it's the suicide in the family home, the bodies under the patio, the baby drowning in the bath. He was no longer the biological specimen I could observe objectively in a medical context, mentally shielded and separated by waterproof apron and visor. He became a familiar scene not just gone wrong, but gone deeply, bottomlessly sad.

§

It's early evening and we're sitting at a table outside in December, beside glowing red heaters and drunk office workers in Santa hats, the temporary Christmas town by the river glittering and lit up around us. We're drinking hot cider, Lara is hiding under a black hood and periodically swigging from a bottle of cough syrup to stave off a winter cold. We've been here for a while. We've talked about our similar Catholic upbringings, how for Catholics death is the event – the thing that all life is working towards – and how the weirdness of such a death-focused religion that keeps severed hands as holy relics can produce people like us. We've talked about how we don't believe in God, how there is probably nothing beyond this, how the human brain struggles to contemplate not existing. And we've talked about the baby. For the last month, I've been emailing her about the baby. I've got more questions about her job, but mostly I just want to talk to someone who was there and saw what I saw. I want to know how she stands it, how she can go back there every day without falling off her feet, and why she would want to. She assures me that this reaction is not unusual – you never know how anyone is going to take it before they get there, whether they have experience with the dead or not. 'It's very circuitous thinking,' she says. 'You wouldn't get into the job if you couldn't handle it, but at the same time, you don't know if you can handle it until you do it.' The actual act of carrying out this job is a mental obstacle for most people, in the beginning. Even her.

'You physically have to move and manipulate people in a way that if you do that to the living, it would hurt them,' she says. She's not just talking about rib shears and bone saws: she's talking about cracking the rigor mortis out of the person's legs, lifting them high above her head just like Sophie did in the embalming room, forcibly snapping them so they would bend. 'I know they're dead, they can't feel this, but it just feels wrong to do it,' she says. 'It's the same with the babies.'

She recalls a baby she had to put back together very early on. She says you can get a better angle on the head stitching if you approach it from the back, but that means turning the baby on its face. She says there's a nicer way of doing it, which is to create a kind of miniature massage table by laying the baby over a sponge, but even so, the first couple of times she did it, it still felt wrong. 'You wouldn't want the parent of this child to see you do this. And when you're washing them, you don't deliberately put a kid's head under water, but…'

Lara is talking faster now, trying to pin down the inherent contradictions of this job that requires both empathy and ruthlessness. In the post-mortem room, before the baby, I had watched her standing over the body of a sixty-something drug addict. Even with the cracking of the rigor he remained curled in the foetal position, his bright green belly keeping to the bend of the curve of his spine, his arm covering it in protection. He was so thin that there were sores where his bones dug into the mattress he'd died on, in a room filled with crack pipes and heroin paraphernalia. He had rings on his fingers, frayed woven bands on his wrists, a single earring and long straggly grey hair. When they opened him up, as well as the APT could do from the side, his lungs were black as tar, adhered to the ribcage. His neck rested on the stand, his empty skull tipped backwards, his mouth open to reveal brown teeth. Lara had paused beside him and said that a case like this makes her wonder what it was like to be him, what it was like to inhabit this body. How did he breathe? What did that feel like? His feet and hands were black with dirt. He was the culmination of years of neglect and malnutrition. When was the last time he shampooed his hair? That day, it was washed and combed for him. Despite the relative brutality of a post-mortem, he was treated with more care by these women than he gave himself.

'... with the baby,' she continues, 'you put him in the tub, you wash him and go grab a towel while leaving him still in the sink full of water, or with his head immersed, and you think *that feels weird*. It's not that it doesn't matter as such, but it's necessary. You *have* to clean this child, and because you can do things you wouldn't do with a living one, you do it because it is easy. The way that you get your job done is completely alien to anything else. It's against anything that you've been taught about what you should do with other people.'

There was a time when Lara did consider working with the living, until someone close to her died. She was studying forensic psychology at university, believing she wanted to work with young offenders, when her friend was murdered – had the shit kicked out of him on a night out by a group of boys and died from a slow bleed on the brain. After that, she no longer believed she had the emotional capacity to help similarly aged offenders, to patiently undo whatever it is that makes someone act out in violence. But why would someone like Lara, who always wanted a job where she would be able to help people, now have a job where she feels like she's hurting them?

She brings up another case, one she says gets to the heart of why she loves what she does. It was a woman in her forties, another drug user, recently relapsed. The family said she had been clean for a long time. 'But people lie, families lie, you never really know.' Everybody figured she had overdosed and the post-mortem was just a formality. But when Lara opened her up, there was not a single organ untouched by cancer. 'No one knew,' she says. 'Absolutely no one knew. Maybe she was in pain, which might explain why she had been using drugs again.' Lara followed the path of the tumour, and found its root in the vicinity of the uterus. 'Gynae cancers can have a strong genetic component, and this woman had children. So we needed to do a lot of testing, and suggested that her family go through genetic counselling.' I think of Terry in his freezer in the Mayo Clinic preparing the lab for practice runs on intricate spinal tumours. Neither he nor Lara can explain why they are not squeamish, or why they can do this every day – Lara doesn't even mind working on the decomposed bodies; she is fascinated by how much people can change, how much life is still going on after death – but both of them have their searchlight on the good it does the living. 'Somebody getting screened for cancer,' she said. 'That was because of me.' She looks, for the first time, proud.

After talking to her for hours, and seeing her at work, it is clear to me what makes Lara able to do this job, and why it would follow on from an abandoned desire to do social work: she is still giving a voice to the voiceless, and her eyes are still drawn to the helpless. Like me becoming overwhelmed by the baby and staying up late to read about infant mortality, what got to Lara at the beginning of her training in the mortuary was the number of dead mothers that came through it – she had no idea just how many dead mothers there are. There is little public discussion about what happens, physically, to a woman after a baby is born – she goes from being a protected vessel to a kind of milk accessory, one so changed physiologically that her post-mortem is a speciality in itself. What shocked Lara was how social factors, like race and economic status, would play such a huge role in whether she lives or dies; Maggie Rae, president of the Faculty of Public Health, was quoted in the British Medical Journal saying that these complex social factors under-lying this increased risk need action beyond the health sector, and long before pregnancy, in order to make any difference. In the days after we speak, Lara sends me piles of information she has kept over the years on maternal deaths. It's not because she wants to be a mother herself, she has no interest in having babies – she tells me she is fuelled purely by feminist rage.

It also upsets her that the role of the APT goes largely unnoticed. It's one that is rarely glimpsed on television – you might see someone in scrubs in the background behind the pretty dead girl on the table, but TV abbreviates the role to the pathologist. Lara didn't know APTs existed until a chance late-night google led her to a blog post written by one. This is pretty much fine and expected – a lot of death is hidden from the public, and TV abbreviates a lot of things for time and money – but it's the fact that the role is also forgotten within the hospital that stings. At an internal event thrown in the wake of the London Bridge attack, to acknowledge and thank the employees for their work in the crisis, Lara recalls a speech given to thank all of the unseen staff. 'Obviously you've got the doctors and the nurses, the frontline staff who deal with this, but then you've got the communications team who had to field tons of phone calls, you have the porters who have to run around the hospital, you have house-keeping, you have catering, you have all these people in these other roles that are important but you never see,' she says, listing everyone who was thanked by job title. But only those who cared for the living were praised from the podium.

'We were not named,' she says, pausing, her perfect eyebrows hovering somewhere near her hairline. She is, still, clearly hurt. 'No one wants praise, no one does this for the glory of it, but you do kind of want some acknowledgement that what you do matters. It matters to the families.'

In the days that followed the speech, Lara says that internal emails announced that all London Bridge patients had left the building (much like Terry at the Mayo Clinic, she calls all of the dead 'patients' even if there was never a time when they were in the building alive, being seen by doctors – they are being cared for by her), along with more thank-yous to everyone for the work they had done. She had stared at the screen dumbstruck, knowing that eight of them were still in her care, waiting to be collected. She resented being forgotten, and she resented the dead being for-gotten too.

'Back in Ancient Egypt, working with the dead was a very, very special profession, whereas now you're reviled. You don't want to say "I love my job" because that makes it sound like you're saying "I'm really happy that your loved one died!"' The smile that is usually so warm is repurposed here as sarcastic and ghoulish. 'But you feel protective over the dead. Kind of like, I will take care of you because no one else will. How do you celebrate work that has essentially come from someone else's pain?'

The emotional burden of this job is not in the taking apart of human anatomy, but the knowledge of what has occurred – the extent of it, the reality of it, the sheer human loss of it. They see the number of babies that lie in their fridges, and because they are the ones that see the totality of it, the APTs here are in support of a formal request to the government to widen coronial jurisdiction to include stillbirths, to find out why so many are dying (the coroner currently only has jurisdiction over deaths if that person breathed outside of their mother). The APTs are among the first to learn the identities of people in mass accidents, and they are among the last to look into the eyes of the people you see in the 'missing' posters. Lara describes walking to work from London Bridge Tube station, in the days after the attack, seeing the faces on the front pages of newspapers and knowing they were in her mortuary. 'I didn't feel like I should be the first one to know this,' she says. 'Not necessarily how they died, but that they are dead. Everyone knows that these people are missing, or that these people are probably dead, but you've got a family who may have a little bit of hope.' She talks about the unidentified suicides that lie in the fridges for days over Christmas, while family members go unnotified because nobody knows their name. 'It feels intrusive, that we know things before the families do.'

The reality of death cannot be denied in the cold, stark light of a hospital mortuary, but attempts are made to mitigate it. There is a viewing room where a pane of glass separates the family from the body, if that is required – usually because of far-gone decomposition, but also in ongoing police cases – though some insist on bypassing the glass to kiss the very dead, while others write them letters they'll never read and stand vigil outside the hospital just to be near. But without the glass between her and the bodies, Lara cannot avoid the truth, and knows – just like in the tarot cards tattooed on her skin – that endings are intrinsically woven into beginnings. This job has solidified what she wants her death to be, but also how she wants to live her life. Her job is to notice things: scars, tumours, the recurring mother's name on another miscarried baby. She notices how many deaths are lonely ones, and mostly she just doesn't want to die forgotten. 'I don't want to be one of the people who lie dead in a flat for months. I want to be missed,' she says. 'I want someone to notice.'

Tough Mother

It's been six months. I still can't stop thinking about the baby in the bathtub. Talking to Lara about what I saw in the post-mortem room helped, but there is still something about it that will not diminish. I keep emailing her; I read everything she sends me about maternal deaths, stillbirths and pregnancy loss. Internet algorithms start assuming this has happened to me – I am, after all, a woman in her mid-thirties – advertising me books on parental grief, leading me to charities and support groups. But it's still not the answer I'm looking for. I'm not grieving – I don't know what I'm doing. Am I traumatised? Probably, but not exactly. It seems bigger than my own internal reaction. I need to speak to someone who understands what I saw – for whom there was no aftermath of personal loss and support groups, just an aftermath of whatever this is.

I remember Ron Troyer, the retired funeral director from Wisconsin, telling me, over a year ago in the cafe, about helping parents dress their dead children. It was another story in a long career of interesting stories when I heard it, but now it kept playing in my mind – how the parents always called the autopsy incision a scar, how he sat with them while they held their cold babies. He had stressed to me the importance of seeing and being with that baby, whether it had lived for months or arrived stillborn, and I had nodded because I had dressed a dead person and agreed that it was an important thing to do. But now it felt like babies were in another category altogether, and that there was another kind of death worker that I had, until this point, not even considered: a midwife.

The role of a midwife, before it became a regulated profession that required medical training, was more of a neighbourly one, as it was across most cultures: they were self-appointed carers during pregnancy and birth. They were also there, before the commercialisation of the funeral industry, to lay out the dead. The bookends of life were considered to be the realm of women. But despite their changed role, there are times when the beginning and the end are the same moment, when babies die before they breathe. Midwives exist at the centre of human power and fragility – they remain life and death workers, both.

I emailed Sands, a stillbirth and neonatal death charity in the UK that I had found in one of my late-night internet searches, and asked them if they would put me in touch with a midwife. I explained what I was doing – that I was writing a book about people who work with death, and that I thought midwives were an overlooked part of that community. They replied within hours, introducing me to a woman whose job I didn't know existed: a bereavement midwife, someone who delivers only the dead or soon-to-be-dead.

Why would a person train for a job so joyful – at least from the outside – only to specialise in its bleakest moments? Did she once feel what I did?

§

In the Heartlands Hospital in Birmingham I get lost on the way to the bereavement ward. Entering the building through the maternity door, I ask a woman on reception for directions. 'Oh love,' she says. 'Bless you.' She gently directs me, soothing like a lullaby, a hand on my back, away from the women resting outdated magazines on the swell of their bellies. I've never had a baby, I'm just someone who came in the wrong door, but you can probably make a good guess about what the issue is with a woman who's hurried in asking for the head bereavement midwife.

When I find her, Clare Beesley wears a blue nurse's outfit with 'MIDWIFE' embroidered on it, black tights and black polished shoes on her small feet. With her blonde hair slicked into a neat beehive, her huge kind eyes and her soft Birmingham accent asking if I'd like a cup of tea, she is almost a cartoon of a caring nurse. I'm anxious and late, but I'm instantly calmed by her presence. I feel like I could tell her anything, like I might accidentally call her Mum. I've known her for twenty seconds.

The ward around us is shades of beige and purple; they've done the best with what the NHS buildings have to offer, and have painted it and filled it with furniture in the most calming colours they could find, though I can imagine this shade of lavender being forever tied in your mind to death. They call it the Eden Ward, and there are autumnal flowers on the doors for each of the three rooms they have here. Clare walks softly into the second one and I follow. She tells me the third is filled with a family, but I never see them or hear them.

It's quiet here on the ward. There's no panic or bustle – it's different from any hospital experience I've had before and every vision of a labour ward I've seen on screen. Clare tells me that they're lucky; in other hospitals women carrying dead babies have to enter the ward through the regular maternity wing, with all the screaming life and hope that comes with new birth. Here, they can come through a side entrance, swerving the mothers whose pregnancies went as planned. Here, when babies are born, there is a silence that is piercing.

We sit on purple chairs on one side of a large bed: a double, with all of the plug sockets and access to oxygen that would come with a regular hospital bed. In the corner, a sink. A clock, a window. There's a coffee table in front of us with a bag of travel-sized toiletries on it, some folded socks, a tube of Polo mints. A typed note says they come courtesy of Sands (the same charity who put us in touch) and that they're for bereaved parents. It's these simple considerations that can count for a lot in strange and awful times. There's a bowl of wrapped cookies and cakes. This feels somewhere between a wellness clinic and a hospital room, as if a hospital room is wearing the wellness clinic's clothes. All of the technical equipment is here – this is a medical environment, after all, and giving birth is physically the same for the mother whether the baby lives or not – but they're trying to ease the blow of why you're in this room: to deliver your dead or almost-dead baby, however small it may be.

Why would anyone be here by choice?

§

As a young midwife Clare was – like many young midwives – unfamiliar with death and unsure of how to deal with it. She still had her grandparents. Nobody in her life had died, other than a pet. When she would see a note on the board in the delivery suite about a family who had lost their baby, she would dread being sent to their side. 'I was so frightened because I knew I couldn't help them,' she says. 'It was really overwhelming to someone who had recently qualified.' (Even now, two decades later, only 12 per cent of neonatal units have mandatory bereavement training.)

About a year into Clare's time as a midwife, a woman went into labour with a baby so young they knew he would not live. He had only been gestating for twenty weeks, which baby growth charts liken to the size of a banana – bigger than a kumquat, smaller than an aubergine. The family were prepared and came with the full knowledge of what was about to happen: that there would be no resuscitation, that twenty weeks was too young for a baby to survive – that notable cases of survival place the foetus's age at a minimum of almost twenty-two weeks. The mother went through her labour knowing there would be no living baby at the end of it, and though he was too young for any medical intervention to save him, when he was born he was breathing.

'Seeing her baby moving and gasping was so distressing for her,' says Clare. 'I just remember, and I won't ever forget it – she was screaming my name. *Clare, you must do something. Please help me. Can't we do something?*' The baby only lived for a few minutes.

When her shift ended, Clare got into her car, shut the door and sobbed. 'I can still feel the emotion I felt at that time. To see someone's raw grief and know that you can't do anything to make that right for them. As somebody who came into a job that everyone perceives as a job of happiness, not the extremes of such devastation and sadness...' She trails off. Now, in the silent ward, she looks like it just happened. Her huge eyes glisten. 'But it's part of your job as a midwife,' she says, visibly steeling herself. 'It's our responsibility.' According to Tommy's – the largest charity carrying out research into pregnancy loss and premature birth in the UK – it is estimated that one in every four pregnancies ends in loss during pregnancy or birth. One in every 250 pregnancies ends in stillbirth; eight babies are stillborn across the UK every day.

A few years later, another midwife set up a bereavement team and asked Clare if she'd like to be part of it. She went along to the training sessions and the more she learned about the situation, the more she realised there was something she could do. She could not breathe life into the baby, but she could look after the families. She couldn't take the situation away, but she could shape it in a way that was less bad. 'I never thought I would lead the service doing this,' she says. 'I came into midwifery to do a happy job, and I've ended up being a bereavement midwife for most of my career. But when you see the difference you can make to parents and their time with their baby, and how that can affect their lives forever, it's such an important part of midwifery. You can't control life events – life isn't in our control – but you can control how you look after a family when they are dealing with the most devastating moment in their lives.'

Clare has been dealing with that moment in strangers' lives for the last fifteen years. Women come here to deliver non-viable foetuses that can fit in the palm of your hand. They come here to deliver full-term babies whose hearts have stopped beating or are not going to survive for very long outside the womb. She sees the concealed pregnancies, the longed-for and doomed pregnancies, the last-ditch attempts fathered by the terminally ill. She sees the relief in women who didn't want a baby in the first place, and she sees parents tear themselves and each other apart over whether or not to carry on despite the severe genetic defect that would only postpone a premature death. She sees mothers and babies die at the same time. She gets in her car at the end of every shift, doesn't turn on the radio, plays no music, and spends the forty-five-minute drive home to her own four children silently decompressing.

§

Clare shows me the cupboard of knitted hats and baby clothes – mostly white, different sizes, from handmade tiny ones to full-term. The knitted caps serve a cosmetic purpose here rather than one of warmth, much like they did in the mortuary with Lara: as a baby passes through the birth canal the planes of its skull overlap so it can fit, but if there is excess fluid in the baby's body – as a result of its death – the planes of the skull can dig into the brain, deforming the head. Clare says she puts a little cap over it and no one can tell the difference. Next to the bonnets are brass-hinged wooden jewellery boxes, or so I think, until she stands on her tip toes to reach one, opens it and it's empty but for a white lace doily. 'These are the coffins for the very little ones,' she says, holding it up so I can see inside.

I had no idea that a bereavement ward existed, let alone coffins for babies as big as my car keys. In my mind I can see the cardboard boxes of all sizes on the trolley in the mortuary at St Thomas' with Lara, many boxes far smaller than the A4 print-out that was balanced on top of each of them for the pathologist. Clare says that there are women who come here who lose their baby at five weeks and react with more devastation to the loss than a woman who loses hers at full term. She says there's no standard emotional weight tied to weeks in the womb. If it's a baby you wanted, it's the loss of potential – an entire other life lived, yours and the baby's, a parallel universe where this didn't happen and other things did, a life that you bought things for, planned things for: clothes, shoes, a pram. It's nothing to do with the size of your baby at all.

'We've all got our own stories behind what happens. You can't say someone who's had a miscarriage at ten weeks is not as important as somebody that's had a stillbirth at term, or a baby that's lived for two days,' she says, placing the wooden box back in the cupboard along-side the others. 'There's so much that's misunderstood about pregnancy loss. The perception that you can just try again makes that little life seem not as important.' I think about the twelve-week rule, how pregnant women are not supposed to say they are pregnant, for fear of jinxing it, for fear of having to say they are no longer pregnant – how that loss is experienced in isolation, expected to be endured in isolation, how for many there is no symbolism, no coffin, and how fewer than half of the women who experience a miscarriage ever find out why it happened. You were an ecosystem, a world with at least one inhabitant, and then you weren't.

We're in the Quiet Room now. This is where family wait for news, as they hover around the tea- and coffee-making facilities. It's where biscuits sit untouched on plates while a baby arrives si-lently in the next room. In the corner is a plastic tree from which paper butterflies hang, labelled with the names of the babies delivered here, with notes from their parents and the scrawled attempts at communication from young siblings.

She opens another cupboard and shows me the stock of memory boxes. They are white, pink, blue. Inside is a blank book for photographs, with space for hand- and footprints. Families are offered a piece of silver jewellery made out of these prints. There is also a box for grandparents, perhaps to mark the moment they became one. Clare says they're working on a pack that they can give to siblings to help them understand what's just happened, to give the baby a place that makes sense in their lives.

Memory boxes are there to record the baby for those who want something they can keep, but they are also there as a safety net for those who aren't sure: families who are too distraught, too afraid to look at their baby because of what they imagine they might see, what image might be indelible in their mind for the rest of time. The midwives can take their baby, photograph it, take prints from their hands and feet, and place these records in a box that can be left unopened, hidden at the back of a closet until one day, years from now, parents might be ready to look. A picture to prove it happened. A footprint to show the baby was tangible. You were someone's mother.

In a 2013 New Yorker piece, Ariel Levy talks about the miscarriage she had at five months on the bathroom floor in a hotel in Mongolia. She held her baby and watched him breathe – a living human, who existed only briefly. She phoned for an ambulance and they told her the baby would not live. 'Before I put down my phone, I took a picture of my son,' she writes. 'I worried that if I didn't I would never believe he had existed … In the clinic, there were very bright lights and more needles and IVs and I let go of the baby and that was the last I ever saw him.' She looked at the photo constantly, and then daily, and it was months before she got it down to once a week. She tried to show the picture to other people, holding her phone up and proving that he was here. Proving to herself, and others, that the baby existed was essential for her to go on living.

Human impulses are the same across centuries – the Victorians needed these photos too, they just took longer to capture. The need in Levy to record was also within the parents standing beside their baby's coffin, waiting for the photographer to signal that it was over.

Memory boxes and photos like Levy's can also be, despite their benign position, a focus of a family's rift. Cracks in relationships can expand to full breaks under such stress – on this ward, people are at their most vulnerable and their most angry – and sometimes there is a push–pull tension where this blank box sits at the middle of the fight. Everybody grieves in their own way, but family members can judge each other on how they do it, can worry if someone is doing it correctly, can step in and try to take charge if they believe they are doing it wrong. The problem with the memory boxes hinges on the fact that people, sometimes, cannot agree on how much time to spend with a dead body, whether it's right to record it, whether they should see the body at all – the crux is the idea that grief can be diminished if you try to forget, or if you literally bury it, just like Spain's Pact of Forgetting. But historical black holes make unsatisfactory graves to bury anything.

How do you move on to grieving if, without the finality of seeing, you're still trapped in disbelief?

Ron Troyer had also told me, when he spoke about helping parents dress their dead children, that it was not uncommon in the past for the father to arrange a swift burial or cremation while the mother was in hospital recovering from the birth – he would make the body disappear so she wouldn't have to see it, and therefore would not become further upset by its presence. It enraged me to hear it: if that happened to me, I would feel like my baby had been stolen from me twice, the second time by someone I could blame. I wondered how many marriages survived it, and if so, for how long. Where did these women put that unspeakable grief and how many were drowned by it?

Clare says this attitude is still not uncommon – in an effort to do good, some people unwittingly do damage. She has, as always, empathy with both sides. 'Your natural instinct is to protect them, isn't it? They don't want to see somebody they love in the pain that they're in, and they think by taking what's happened away, it takes the pain away. But it doesn't.'

In some of Clare's cases, I struggle to imagine the reasoning behind the things these people do. She recalls one family where the very dominant father was adamant he did not want a memory box, but the meek mother, in a quiet word to the midwives, revealed she very much did. The midwives secretly made her one, recording the body of her baby in photograph and footprint, and smuggled it into her bag as she was leaving the hospital. Three months later, she phoned the ward in tears: he had found the box and destroyed it.

'It may be him not being able to cope with seeing that,' says Clare. 'It may be him finding it upsetting that his wife's upset by seeing that. But we don't store photos, because we're not legally allowed to. We didn't have anything that we could give her back. That was gone forever.'

I ask her if this reticence to engage with the body of the baby is present at the scene of its birth. Do people always want to see their baby? Or do some place a block between them, mentally regard it as some biological malfunction to be removed and forgotten?

I can hear Poppy the funeral director saying, 'The first dead body you see should not be someone you love.' I imagine the events of seeing a dead body for the first time and having your baby die twinned in the one moment and I feel sick. I wonder how much the fear of the unknown, a desperate act of self-preservation, robs parents of their one chance to meet their baby.

'In the majority of cases most people do want to see the baby,' she says. 'Initially, not always, but when the baby's born, they do. It's about preparation. Seeing a baby that's born at twenty weeks is very different to a baby that's born at term. They're quite shiny. They do look different, in terms of their skin colour, their transparency. And I think everyone googles after a doctor's appointment, don't they? They can't help themselves.'

Babies die for many reasons, and some of those reasons are visible: here they deliver babies with severe abnormalities, from major spina bifida, where the spinal cord is not enclosed within the skin, to anencephaly, a defect of the brain and skull, where the top of the head just isn't there. Then there are the babies whose hearts have stopped beating but the induction has been slow (because the mother's body hasn't responded to the medication, or for some other reason) and the baby has stayed where it is for days, maybe weeks. Within or without the womb, dead bodies change: the colours turn, the skin peels. Clare says the skin can look like a blister, bright red underneath. 'That's upsetting for families because their instant reaction is, Is that painful?' The parents aren't sure if it happened while the baby was still living. 'It isn't painful. It's just where the fluid isn't circulating around the body any more, so it seeps under the skin. It makes the skin very fragile.'

To all of my questions about the reactions of parents, Clare keeps saying that everyone is different, that there is no one correct way of reacting to your dead baby, and there is no one way that people do. We are squeamish, as a society, about dead bodies; we're conditioned to be apart from them. We construct them in our imaginations, stacking them up to all the heights of horror our minds are capable of. To have one come out of you, and then to hold it, is another experience entirely. Clare tries to work out the best approach for each family. If a family is very unsure, she will offer the baby in stages and ease them into it gradually. She will take the baby away, spend time with him, then come back and tell them how he looks. She may suggest looking at photographs first. She might wrap their baby in a blanket completely, or have their tiny feet poke out the end for them to hold. Most families, treated gently and with as much time as they need, end up changing their minds.

'I think people are almost relieved, in a way, that it isn't what they built in their mind. It's almost like, *Oh my gosh, she looks like a baby*. Of course she does. She's your baby. The one thing that I've become a lot more confident in is that you just have to be kind – always kind – but honest,' she says, 'and very sensitive in what you say and how you say it. If parents aren't shocked by what they see, it's because you've done your job. You've prepared them. It's a hard thing for a parent to say, "Actually, I am frightened about seeing my baby." It's about normalising some of their feelings in these circumstances. None of it feels normal, and to the outside world, none of it is normal.'

The benefit of the bereavement ward is that nobody is hiding death from you, so you know the full breadth of what you're allowed to do – which is, essentially, anything you feel you need to. It isn't like this everywhere: in a study by the University of Michigan, published in 2016, they found that of the 377 women spoken to whose babies were stillborn or died soon after birth, seventeen were told by doctors and nurses that they could not see their baby at all, and thirty-four were refused when they asked to hold them. The study was to investigate the level of PTSD and depression in bereaved mothers, but they were unable to draw conclusions on whether or not holding your baby had an effect on the four-fold likelihood of depression, or the seven-fold higher odds of PTSD, since so many reported they did not get the chance. But they did find that what Clare said was true: that it didn't matter if your baby was born dead, or if they lived for a few days. The mental and emotional wake of baby loss has nothing to do with the baby's age.

On the bereavement ward, seeing is grieving. Mothers who have been focusing purely on getting through the physical side of the process will know that should they want to hold their baby, they can. If she knows her baby won't be resuscitated, she can hold her baby to her heart as the smaller heartbeat fades. Whatever they want to do, Clare will be there with them to assist and facilitate.

'You'll never know those options if you haven't had somebody discuss it all with you,' says Clare. 'How would you even imagine seeing your dead baby, let alone thinking, *Do I want hand and footprints or do I want photos or do I want to hold my baby while my baby dies?* How do you even think about all these things? The hardest thing for families is looking back and having regrets. In years to come, thinking, *I had a chance to hold my baby and I didn't.*'

§

The summer before I arrived late at the bereavement ward, the news was full of pictures of a whale: an orca still carrying her dead calf with her, ten days after its death, pushing it with her head as she swam through waters off British Columbia. After seventeen months of gestation, she had been somebody's mother for thirty minutes. Finally, the whale let go, and that made the news too. She had tired herself out in the cold sea, pushing the weight of her grief.

We look to whales as avatars of human emotion. We can't help it; they are so unknown, mysterious and vast that we can project anything we like onto them as if they are the side of a building, an emotional Rorschach test. The orca made the news because she wouldn't let her dead baby go: we were collectively heartbroken for her, though it was weird, some thought, that she pushed this corpse with her through the ocean when she could swim off and forget. There she was, rising from the deep, dragging something from our subconscious and showing it to us on the news, telling us that pretending it didn't happen is not the same as grieving. While nobody can measure or predict anyone's grief when a person of any age dies – people mean things to us that are ours to feel uniquely – baby loss is its own realm. You're losing someone you thought you had, who no one is going to meet, so your loss is unshareable except to the few who were there. Whale or human, some cannot let the body go because it's all they have.

The mortuary here on the Eden Ward is theirs alone: no babies lie wrapped on trays below adults, there is no designated refrigerator in a vast wall of refrigerators in the basement of a hospital. Here they have just the one, in a room painted sky blue, with a mural of small flowers in pink and lavender. Far from the stark fluorescence of other hospital mortuaries, it is one you can sit and spend time in. Some parents return every day until the funeral to read the baby stories. Some phone the ward in the middle of the night, unable to sleep, and ask that someone check on their baby. Others take their baby home in a small cot fitted with a cooling unit, and try to cram a lifetime into the two weeks they have before the funeral, before the ground or the crematorium takes their tiny body away – they have picnics with the basket beside them, the baby's older siblings playing nearby. Some push their babies in crisp new prams to the garden behind this building. It too has a tree – a real one, this time – decorated in the fluttering names of the many babies who passed through here.

Baby death is something we don't know how to talk about: miscarriages go unspoken, news of a stillbirth is often met with stunned silence. Nobody wants to say the wrong thing, so nobody says anything. New parents, without their babies, become part of a club they never signed up for, invisibly exiled in the crowd. Lives never go back to the way they were. Which is why, in a senior role that could easily become an administrative one, Clare insists on remaining clinical. She wants to be someone who was there in the room, she wants to be one of the few who met this baby, someone the families can come back to years later if they are emotionally lost, or if they are pregnant again and want to speak to someone who understands the fragility of their body and mind, someone who understands their very real fear of things going wrong again. Clare has seen the fear and she has felt it: in her own fourth and final pregnancy, something was wrong – her baby had stopped growing, and she knew the reality of everything that might be coming. Her husband – who she describes as not an emotional man at all – had seen her dread, her quiet worry, and cried when the baby arrived safely, after an emergency C-section. She admits she is wildly overprotective as a mother, and fears death only because her children would be without her. She has seen it happen time and time again on the ward.

As I leave, somewhat dazed, Clare points me in the direction of the small garden. I walk around the pebble path and look back at the plain brick building from this self-conscious oasis, carved out of the middle of a cement hospital block, tended by volunteers. I read the names on the plastic butterflies as they catch the light. I wonder what the baby in the bathtub was called, whether it would help, if I knew it, to write his name here. 'Do something,' the woman had pleaded with Clare, holding her tiny, gasping baby, all those years ago. '*Do something.*' I think about Clare sobbing in her car, and I think about the baby in the bath, how I stood and watched him sink, how I could not make him live and I could not make it better, and I remember how I wanted – more desperately than I have ever wanted anything – to do something. The pinwheels in the flowerbeds spin in the breeze. If you look up you can see the windows of the rooms where the babies arrive into Clare's waiting arms.

Earth to Earth

It's early spring. The trees still mostly bare, the clouds heavy and dark. Small clumps of yellow primrose flowers pop up between the unruly graves. Arnos Vale, a cemetery built in Bristol in 1837, is a place now filled with headstones swallowed by ivy, where thick roots lift grave markers and topple them sideways so they lean on their neighbours. I like this about old Victorian graveyards: they are not the obsessively tidy visions of Los Angeles cemetery parks, with lawns mowed to golfing-green perfection and marble headstones shining and white. Those are a display of constant battle against the encroachment of nature, while cemeteries like this are places of death overtaken by the relentless force of life, and moss. Graves are engulfed by vines and leaves as if in an embrace of ownership. Death is part of life, they say. Death is part of all of it.

I flinch a bit as I pass a teddy bear with its head pulled off, its back slumped against a cross that has fallen off its base, and walk further up the steep hill. This will be a much easier interview than the autopsies and the bereavement midwife, I hope. I'm still feeling raw. Being outside, instead of in a hospital ward or basement mortuary, helps.

At the uppermost point of the cemetery, by the Cross of Sacrifice and Soldier's Corner, where forty sailors have lain since they lost their lives in World War Two, all I can hear is birds. There I find Mike and Bob looking out through the windscreen of the muddiest van that ever existed. Bob is sixty, with few teeth and straggly dark hair that hangs down as if his head sprouted it from one central point. His face is disappearing into his shoulders and hoodie, like an egg in an egg cup. Mike, seventy-two, the speaker for the both of them, hops out of the van and waves me up the brow of the hill, shouting in his strong Bristolian accent that I was mad and I should have driven. His neat white hair is shaved at the sides, and the closer I get, the more visible the dusting of dirt on his jeans and navy blue fleece becomes. 'Do you want to see what we've done, then?' He's smiling, instantly friendly. Bob waves sweetly from his seat in the van and mimes that he wants to stay where it's warm. Mike walks me over uneven ground to the open grave.

Thick, green fabric has been laid around its grassy edges. Two long planks of wood lie at the sides of the hole for stability when the pallbearers come to stand there. More green fabric is laid on top of those, draping into the hole, lining walls that are so crisp that the cut planes of roots align with the clay as if sliced by a machine. Two thinner pieces of wood are placed across the grave in a V shape, waiting to bear the coffin while the vicar reads the words of committal before it is lowered, on woven canvas straps looped around the handles, into the dirt. The mound of excavated soil is piled next to the hole, covered with more green fabric. There is no visible loose soil, apart from right at the bottom – a thin buffer between the husband who's already in there and the wife whose funeral is currently happening a little way down the road. Mike says you can tell when you're getting close to the existing coffin in a family plot – the soil tends to be a bit wetter, or if it's a particularly old grave, the lid can cave in.

I look down. There, past my coat flapping around my knees, my boots an inch from the edge, is the void. I've stood here before, under a strung-up tarpaulin in a flat, treeless Australian cemetery, holding my grandfather's hand as I watched my grandmother's coffin being sealed into a cement vault above ground. She had always been vocally and specifically scared of decaying six feet below – something about the worms frightened her more than oblivion (she was a Catholic). Standing there then, I had wondered if she would bake in the summer heat, locked in her cement box.

It turns out there is a strange disconnect standing over the open grave of someone I don't know. I'm not holding someone's hand trying to process news. My thoughts are not clouded with the loss of a person in my life, there are no memories shooting through the projector in my mind of things that won't happen again, and I cannot imagine the person as they might look now, or as they might look six months from now, because I've never seen their face. I look into that grave and all I think about is me: what it would feel like to lie there and look up, to see myself looking down from the lip of it.

Mostly I think it looks cold down there. I remember another thing Ron Troyer told me, that when you die in the American Midwest in winter, your body won't be buried until the spring, when the ground has thawed enough to dig – until then, you take up space in a mausoleum, beside temporary neighbours. But occasionally, he said, farmers would insist on a winter burial: they worked in the mills and knew exactly how cold a building above ground could get, and how much warmer it was six feet down. The gravediggers, lured by Ron's promises of bourbon, would drag out their charcoal cookers – a sort of grave-length metal dome – and leave them there for twenty-four hours, defrosting the frozen ground so they wouldn't break their mechanical diggers. Opening a grave in a Midwestern winter is like trying to dig in cement.

The soil here, below me, is mostly clay, and Mike says it's one of the best places to dig; the clay provides a natural structural integrity that thinner soils don't, so it won't cave in when you're halfway down. He and Bob cover most of the burial grounds in this area and have done since they left school. He says the locals call them Burke and Hare.

Tucked behind the mound of excavated earth, sitting on the corner of the green fabric, is a small, brown, urn-shaped pot with a cork lid. It's battered with indents of wear and age, and covered in muddy fingerprints that have been haphazardly wiped away. Mike uncorks it and holds it up for me to see, explaining that it's the soil for the vicar to throw as he's committing the body to the ground, doing the 'ashes to ashes, dust to dust' bit. I notice that it's a different soil to the kind inside the grave or heaped beside it – it's drier, but it's also finer. It's closer to sand than the clay that came out of the hole. I ask him if it came from here, or if he got it elsewhere. 'Molehills,' says Mike, pushing the cork back in. He collects them in his garden, scoops them into the pot to have on hand for the vicar: the finer soil kicked up by the feet of moles lands softer on the lid of a coffin than a lump of clay. 'It's always nice soil in a molehill,' he says, tucking it back behind a headstone.

§

Some of the world's most famous architecture, our most beloved wonders, are graves. The pyramids of Egypt. India's Taj Mahal. Monuments built to house the dead. There are few things that I can think of where the difference between basic and luxury is so great than in what you do with a dead body. What could be more basic than a hole in the ground? More grand than the Taj Mahal?

We're in the formerly white van now, eating the wine gums that Mike keeps in a freezer bag on the dashboard for the pallbearers. He cracked them open when he asked me to guess how old I thought he was and I landed on a number twelve years younger than he actually is, which tickled him so much he keeps bringing it up, even to Bob, who was there when I said it. We haven't moved since. He's in the driver's seat, I'm in the passenger seat, and Bob's squashed between us, shoulder to shoulder, forming one multiheaded mass, a wine gum-eating hydra. The footwell is caked with thick mud that I'm assured is less of a problem in summer. We're staring out, chewing, waiting for the funeral cortege. Mike and Bob do this with every funeral: the grave is not finished until you fill it, and they want to make sure everything goes right. They won't make themselves obvious, but they will linger in the surroundings until they are needed, which can be earlier than usual if an overzealous pallbearer lowers the coffin like a submarine diving below. Mike will step in, briefly, to even out the angle.

While we wait, Mike tells me how to dig a grave. Bob adds mostly unintelligible giggles that Mike translates, and when he laughs we feel it, so squashed are we in the cabin. Mike says you need to know the dimensions of the person before you break the ground, but people tend to underestimate out of politeness, so they habitually dig it wider than suggested so nobody gets wedged or stuck – it's happened in the past, when coffin handles have jutted out a little further than expected and more digging was required while the family milled around in shoes not made for marshy ground. A family plot for six people needs to be ten feet deep, while a smaller one for three or less only needs to go down six, and the coffin at the top of the stack is covered with a paving slab to keep animals out. If the area isn't too overgrown or crowded with headstones, they use a mini mechanical digger for most of the job – a sort of mobility scooter with a long arm that lives on a small trailer behind the van. Bob operates the digger while Mike directs, running out ahead of the machine to lay wooden boards like railway tracks to protect the grass. But if they can't get the digger into the area, they do it all by hand: just men and shovels and physical labour. It can take a whole day to dig a grave by hand. In old churchyards, they occasionally find bones where there are no markers, where the coffin has disappeared around the body. They bag up the bones and put them back in the ground. Nobody leaves the place they were buried.

There comes a point in the digging process when you have to get inside the grave to finish it. For that, they have a rotating cast of young men, students who pass the job onto others as they find new ones, or when summer holidays end. The walls of the grave that I noticed were so neat, with the roots trimmed so deliberately, are only that way because some young guy got in and straightened the walls that surrounded him. It's his feet that occasionally feel the lid of the coffin give way.

Mike and Bob have buried friends, babies, murder victims that later needed to be exhumed, and both of them have buried their mothers – they helped each other dig them, like they would any other grave. When they themselves die, those graves will be reopened and their coffins placed a couple of inches above the lids of their mothers'. They have both, already, dug and stood inside their own graves. When I ask what that feels like, they glance at each other. They don't think about it too much. Mike says that death, like a grave, is just a practical thing: you're an outsider looking in, even if you're standing in it. And why would anyone else dig the grave when they're the local gravediggers? They'd do the same job for anyone, whether it's a mother or a stranger. Bob says he's just looking forward to being with his mum again, having lived with her all his life until she died two years ago. But he's frightened of the graveyard at night. 'She'll look after me,' he mumbles, smiling shyly.

The wine gums are passed around again. We hear the horses first – the clip-clop of their hooves – and then, through the dirty windscreen, we can see their plumes in the distance.

§

The coachman in his top hat pulls the ornate black carriage to the side of the road, the coffin of the wife half obscured by the abundance of wreaths in the back. Mike has jumped out of the van to help direct the pallbearers where to go, the only man not in a suit yet somehow making himself almost invisible. He stands among the graves, head bowed, hands clasped in front of his muddy fleece, waiting. He says that sometimes mourners notice him and ask questions. How long will the coffin last? Will worms eat my father? He tells them worms don't go down that far: they're physically able to, but generally they stay closer to the surface – six feet is too deep for them to bother. Mostly everything mourners want to know is worm-related. I think of my grandmother in her above-ground grave and I believe him.

I loiter behind the vicar's bright red Vauxhall, away from the family. Bob stays in the van. Four pallbearers carry the coffin to the wooden stand at the foot of the grave, take a moment to reconfigure themselves, then move it to the planks that suspend it above the opening. Mike is behind the vicar now, a few graves over, hands clasped again, head bowed. His small pot of soft, dry molehills is beside the vicar's feet. He stands there for the whole ceremony, always watchful of when he might need to leap in and help, and eventually he does: standing between the suits, grabbing a strap, lowering the coffin into the ground, slowly, then retreating again.

It's 3.45 p.m., and children are walking home from school through the cemetery. Over the monotone of the vicar reading the final words of committal, children scream at each other that someone has died. The coachman, still clutching the reins of the horses, grimaces awkwardly.

The mourners leave, holding each other's arms as they pick their way through the old graves, and the gravediggers get to work. Bob slides out of the van, and Ewan – today's young help – appears from wherever it is he's been all this time. Planks are picked up, fabric is folded and stacked in a wheelbarrow. Bob unloads the mini digger from the trailer while Mike re-lays the boards over the imprints in the grass. Ewan shovels in a layer of dirt by hand so that when the digger comes there will be a cushion between the heavy, falling clay and the wooden lid of the coffin. Bob scoots over in his fun-size machine and pushes the mound of earth back into the hole while the other two tidy the edges and place the wreaths on top of the grave. Holly, pink roses, daffodils. Shovels, left to the side while other work is going on, stick into the ground and lean against each other for support.

The diggers stand back and consider their work. They're disappointed there's no marker to put back at the head of the grave to finish it off. Mike figures that maybe the family was waiting until the death of the next person before having one made. The man had lain in an unmarked grave for years, waiting for his wife.

Soil subsides and changes with seasons and rain, so any leftover earth is used to top up uneven graves in the area. Mike collects the clumps of clay that have rolled into the nearby sailors' headstones and looks around for graves whose surfaces could do with evening out, filling the hollow parts with what he has to hand. All the tools and equipment are tidied and packed up in less than half an hour. The gravediggers are back in their van, waving from the window as they head out, Bob once again shrinking into his hoodie.

There is so much trust in a burial. You are entering a piece of land outside of your control. What happens to it after you are buried depends on other people. Whether the grass is trimmed, the ground above you sinks or headstones are left to topple. Whether the entire acre of land is sold or transformed, or your bones moved to make way for a railway tunnel. Being buried is an act of blind faith. You have no idea. You are just being left there, in a box, with no minders. But here there is someone keeping an eye on you as they pass, topping up the sunken bits, wondering where your headstone is. And when the vicar threw the molehills from the pot, it was true they landed like feathers.

The Devil's Coachman

Tony Bryant has saved a coffin for me. I'm forty-five minutes late because of a cancelled train and I'm running up the path when I see him standing out the front, waiting, the blocky brick crematorium chapel looming behind him. He's in his mid-fifties, wearing a tight black T-shirt tucked in to black jeans and a studded leather belt. Faded tattoos poke out the bottom of his sleeves. In his thick West Country accent he shouts, 'We've co-ordinated our outfits!' Mine is sweatier. Dragging myself up hills while Bristolian men wave at me from afar seems to be my MO now.

Through a door around the back of the building, we head down the grey and green linoleum stairs, all edged in yellow-and-black-striped hazard tape, to the basement. A wooden coffin sits on a white steel hoist in front of four furnaces, each with their own metal door. A printed photograph of two young blonde children is tucked under the engraved metal nameplate next to the green floral clay that once held the wreath in place in the chapel upstairs.

It really doesn't matter that I've now seen coffins, empty, standing in rows in a mortuary, or others, occupied, in funeral homes. There is a symbolism and a reality in a coffin that still winds me. I've sat at intersections waiting for the lights to change, then missed it because a hearse drove by, brought back from my thoughts by beeps and horns. In my mind I'm picturing it: the shoulders aligned in the angled corners, the lid so close to the nose, the hands holding each other in the dark. Seeing a coffin in a stark industrial setting like this, denuded of flowers and religious ceremony, is a different kind of shock from seeing the hearse and car pull up outside your house to take you and your family to the church – but the power this box holds is still there.

Tony walks around the coffin and motions to me to follow him, ducking through the gap between the machines to get to the touchscreen controls: unexpectedly high-tech for something made of fire and brick yet still designed with a similar aesthetic to Windows 95 (before the touchscreen he had a manual control board with buttons he describes as being like Doctor Who's TARDIS). Nearby, tubs of ashes line two shelves against the brick wall. Tony tells me they belong to families waiting to decide if they want to witness the scattering of the ashes – the ones on the top are for people who have already decided they don't want to be there for it, but he gives them two weeks to change their minds. Some do. In a small office off the cremating room, he keeps those that are waiting to be collected. Sometimes, no one comes for them.

The temperature of the space inside the bricks needs to be 862 degrees Celsius so it will incinerate, not cook. We stand at the screen and watch the numbers flick over: 854, 855. A bar graph in the middle shows the levels of various things and Tony explains them over the loudening roar. I catch bits of it, something about the cooling and heating and filtering of air so that there's no visible smoke outside the building. He's pointing at a spaghetti junction of steel pipes above us, compartments below us. He's explaining UV sensors, air flow, spark plugs. He opens the hatch to the main burner – the heart of the machine, the fire that heats the furnaces. The flames rage, burning the fresh oxygen as it rushes in to feed them. A black beetle scuttles past on the floor, its long articulated body raised in a curl behind it like a scorpion. I point at it. 'That's called a Devil's Coachman!' Tony shouts above the noise, grinning because he knows I won't believe him. I google it later and it's true.

The numbers march on: 861, 862. Tony rushes back through the walkway, where the coffin is waiting by the doors to the furnaces. He tells me to stand back in the corner where I won't get in the way, and presses a blue button. One door slides up to reveal a glowing orange oven lined with bricks, and a cement floor as ravaged as the surface of the moon. I squeeze myself into the corner and can still feel the heat on my face from ten feet away.

'This is very unceremonious,' he says, his hand on the foot of the coffin.

Here is a fact that only becomes obvious when you're standing in front of an open cremator: there are no wheels on the bottom of a coffin. There are no pulleys or levers to gently move this heavy object from the hoist to the hot place where it will ultimately disappear – at least, there aren't any in this crematorium. And so there's this: the unceremony of Tony relying on momentum and aim alone. He slides the coffin back on the smooth metal hoist and then charges it, one-armed, with all of his weight, into the mouth of the oven. My involuntary gasp is lost in the roar as the coffin rumbles across the uneven cement. Sparks fly and glitter white against the orange. The picture of the children flutters to a corner and combusts. The coffin is already on fire as the door comes down. I step forward to look through the peephole and watch as it is swallowed by flames. There's a faint smell of steamed clams.

Tony holds his arms out to show me: one bigger than the other, a lopsided Popeye. 'I should swap sides occasionally, I suppose,' he says, laughing. Why change a habit of thirty years?

§

Canford Crematorium in Bristol averages about eight bodies a day, maybe 1,700 a year. Tony walks up from his lodge inside the cemetery (it comes with the job) and turns the machine on at seven o'clock every morning, giving it a couple of hours to preheat before the first cremation. They've had four already this morning, and three scheduled for this afternoon. I'm here in the quiet gap between them. Tony keeps checking his watch.

The cemetery that surrounds this place is about a hundred years old, the crematorium half of that. Since the time it was built, the cremation rate in the UK has risen from around 35 per cent to 78 per cent of all funerals (America is lagging behind at 55 per cent). The size of people has changed too: if you're over six foot ten, or weigh over 150 kg, it is possible your coffin won't fit through the hole in the floor of the old chapel that allows your body to be transported downstairs. Local funeral homes are aware of this and take larger clients elsewhere.

Before Tony got the job in the basement, he worked outside as one of twelve gardeners, tending to the thirty rose beds and some 2,000 bushes, trimming the hedges and shrubbery, keeping watch over the greenhouse that grew fresh flowers for the chapel vases that are now filled with plastic displays. But the machinery of cremation interested him, the money was (marginally) better, and, he said, 'You can't stay outside getting cold and wet forever.' Downstairs, you're always warm.

We're in the kitchen now, the kind of bare governmental back room that is made only slightly less bleak by comedy signs about quitting your job and the kind of mugs that are left behind after Secret Santas and Easter eggs. One has Homer Simpson holding Spider Pig up to the ceiling, and Tony is drinking black instant coffee from it. His colleague, Dave, is eating toast with ham and fried eggs. Dave's black suit jacket hangs on a hook by the door, his matching black tie tucked inside his shirt so he doesn't get egg on it before the funeral service. He's younger than Tony, about my age, with dark hair and a goatee beard. When I meet him he's reading a copy of Dracula he found on the wall outside someone's house. There are supermarket chocolate-chip muffins in a plastic tray on the Formica table. We eat them while bodies downstairs burn in their furnace cubicles.

I'm here at the crematorium to see the industrial end of death: the part where all of the ceremony and courtesy of dealing with the living has passed and bodies are consumed by flames. I've met people who organise funerals, another who carefully takes imprints of faces, and someone who meticulously sets those features for the family's final look. This is the place beyond that, the basement, where the interaction with the living is over and all we have is men moving coffins to ovens, and bones to blenders. Or at least that's what I thought, but I very quickly realise that's not exactly the case.

I've been talking to them for an hour and what has struck me the most is the disconnect between what happens above and what happens below, how a lack of knowledge in what happens in death – either by general ignorance or funeral directors not being straight with people – leads to things going wrong, or less well, downstairs. Tony says he never would have taken a job that involved touching dead bodies – 'They're spooky, innit' he says, recoiling – and mostly, he doesn't have to. If everyone was more aware of how the system works, dead bodies would remain only the theoretical contents of a sealed box. But a family arguing for months about who's going to pay for the now much-delayed funeral doesn't think of the man in the crematorium when the body finally arrives. They don't picture Tony, waiting, his back against the wall in the furthest corner of the basement, listening to the final notes of the organ as the mourners leave, already able to smell what is about to come down on his hydraulic lift. They don't think ahead to the body leaking and contaminating the hearse, the chapel and finally the basement, engulfing him in a funk of decay for days – a stench so bad the funeral director apologetically gifted him air freshener that, according to Tony, smelled even worse than the dead man. 'Have a go on that,' he says now, incredulously, holding up the small brown bottle he's fetched from his office, the lid already off. It smells like chemical liquorice. I agree it would be olfactory warfare to put this in a diffuser. 'There's a time limit on a dead body,' he says, screwing the lid back on tightly. 'Sometimes I think funeral directors skirt round it.' He puts the bottle back on a shelf, never to be used.

Then there's the funeral directors selling coffins made of wicker or cardboard, pitching them as a greener alternative to families who want to do environmental good. When they originally entered the market, nobody considered the physical action of 'charging' a coffin, and how much of that relied on solid wood being able to skate across cement. Early designs would combust and vanish before the coffin was all the way in – leaving crematorium staff to push the body into the cremator without it. Now, after much discussion and testing, they come with a solid board base. But the wood from a traditional coffin also serves as fuel for flames, so to compensate for its absence Tony has to turn on the gas jets – transforming the coffins into not quite the eco-friendly alternative they were sold as. Without combustion, the body merely bakes. Peer through the peephole and it looks like a man in a wetsuit. The jets blast the body apart.

In response to whether thirty years of this makes him think about his own death, or his own body being burned, Tony is proudly showing me pictures of his dog, Bruno: a white and speckled-brown rescue Staffie, his huge tongue lolling out of his beefy face. Tony is beaming like a man in love. 'I missed it! I escaped my own death!' he says, so far failing to explain why I'm looking at a picture of a dog, not that I mind. 'I got run off the back of me motorbike at 60 mph, four years ago. Old Bruno was in the sidecar.' As Tony's head hit the ground, Bruno sailed on unharmed in the sidecar of the Kawasaki Drifter, eventually coming to a stop a little further down the road. Tony ended up in hospital, while Bruno sat patiently in his stationary seat, waiting to be collected.

Tony regularly gives tours of the place, much like I'm getting today, to new vicars or funeral directors so they have more of an idea of what actions above mean to those below – but the thing that's becoming increasingly clear is that this job isn't confined purely to the basement, or even to the dead. Sometimes those tours are given to the dying, who are planning their own funeral and want to know exactly what will happen. Tony will show them the catafalque in the chapel – the decorative plinth that bears the coffin, with its hidden industrial lift controlled by a brass button in the pulpit, worn and discoloured by decades of celebrant fingers – and tell them they have a choice of whether or not they would like it lowered at the end of the service. (Most don't. Partly, this is because of the misconception that the coffin is being lowered directly into flames. Others want to say goodbye to the coffin in their own time; having a vicar press a button means you only get as long as their schedule allows you. 'One time a vicar collapsed and pressed the button accidentally and we had to send it back up,' says Dave, laughing. 'We had to get another vicar to finish the

service off. It was food poisoning, apparently. He just flaked out.')
Tony will show them the religious options and the less so, like the
curtains that can be pulled in front of the crosses to obscure them.
Sometimes he sits upstairs to fill a pew at the council-funded
cremations for the poor or forgotten who had no mourners of
their own, always in the 9.30 a.m. slots that are harder to sell. Tony
and Dave make sure everyone has someone at their funeral, even if
it's just the two of them.

For the last five years or so Dave has been the substitute for
every role in the building: he covers the crematorium downstairs
when Tony's away, he's the chapel attendant on other days, he occasionally digs graves or steps in to carry a coffin if a pallbearer is
looking a little wobbly on their feet. He even scatters ashes in the
cemetery, performing small intimate ceremonies for the families.
He says that standing there at the chapel door, looking at the backs
of all these mourners' heads, he finds it impossible not to picture
who might fill the seats at his own funeral one day. But what gets to
him, mostly, is being around bereaved people eight hours a day: he
gets empathy fatigue from seeing people so sad all the time and
knowing he cannot help, or can only help in a finite way. Vicars,
in their training, are taught to take some time out after a funeral
to recharge – but Tony and Dave go on to the next, and the next.
They sit in the pews, or stand at the doors, or wait for the coffins
downstairs. And while funerals end after an hour or so, cemeteries
do not.

'Because I work here, people ask me if I believe in ghosts,' says
Dave. 'I categorically do not believe in ghosts, but you do see ghosts
every day in this place. It's the people who are visiting, day after
day, and they're alive and kicking but they're so bereaved that all
they've got left is coming here and going to the gravestone and
standing there.'

Dave tries to befriend them, these ghosts, when he's out in the
cemetery tending to the grounds. There's the guy with the deck-
chair and the newspaper. The mother and son who do a lap of the
cemetery daily and read the Quran at the bottom of the garden.
But it's the widowers he struggles with: the old men who travel up

on the bus and stand alone in the wind or rain. He says he can't help but create stories about them, imagining a nagging guilt in the man who buys his dead wife expensive flower arrangements three times a week that Dave, days later, has to put in the bin. It eats at him. He suddenly looks exhausted just talking about it. 'Eventually you end up avoiding them, because you know they're going to suck the life out of you just by saying hello.'

It goes quiet in the kitchen, and Tony pushes the muffins across the table at me with his bigger arm. He asks if it doesn't get *me* down, hanging around in places like this for whatever it is I'm doing – it was explained to him, vaguely, down the chain of character references that led me here, but it was hard to elaborate over the sound of the machine. I tell him that 'down' isn't really how I'd put it. I tell him that some things get to me in a way that others don't, but I stop short of telling him about the baby. I tell him that I think the difference is that I'm a visitor in this world and can leave at any time, so what sticks is not the sadness – which, as Dave said, can be cumulative – but the stories of people doing the good and right thing even though no one will notice. From Terry swapping the faces back in the Mayo Clinic, to the funeral director sneaking in exiled boyfriends after hours to say goodbye during the AIDS crisis in small-town America, to the gravedigger and his feather-light molehills. There is tender care here, if you look for it. So many of these jobs, like Tony and Dave's, aren't limited to the text in the advert.

§

'This is an example of a perfect cremation,' says Tony, standing in front of the machine, finger poised at the button.

He opens the metal door and I peek inside. We're at the other end of the machine, the opposite to where we stood when he charged the coffin. If the body were still there, we would be at the head, looking down at the feet, but it only takes a couple of hours for a coffin and person to be reduced to a smouldering pile of bones and charcoal. The coffin is gone now. The back of the skull has been crushed under the weight of itself – all bones

become more fragile, like 3D dust. Still visible are the perfectly intact structures of the eye sockets, nose and forehead, surrounded
by glowing embers of wood burning themselves into oblivion.
Beyond the skull, delicate ribs, a pelvis, just one full femur, the
bones scattered inside the machine, having been moved by air
and fire from the positions they once held in the body. A young,
fit person will have a stronger, harder skeleton to leave behind,
but this was an old woman – osteoarthritis weakens bones before flames do. When Tony touches them with a long metal rake,
they break apart. The skull collapses and the face disappears, as if
below waves.

'Right, do you want to rake this one down or what?' he says.

Tony hands me the rake and directs me on how to use it. Like
playing pool in a cramped pub, it has maybe six inches of clearance
before it hits the wall behind us – something Tony has gotten used
to in time, but I keep hitting the brick. Right to left, left to right.
The sound of metal dragging on cement is thunderous, adding to
the roar of the burner. He points out the metal roller at the front
of the oven that I can rest the handle on and suddenly everything
is easier on my back. The heat has lowered considerably since the
coffin went in, but my skin feels close to burning by being so
near. I'm finding it hard to get all the pieces, with the bumps
and crevasses in the floor of the cremator, the effects of time and
wear – the floor of their more recently restored cremator is comparatively smooth. Tony grabs a smaller, more delicate rake and
takes over, making sure each piece and pile of ash goes down the
hole at the front of the machine to cool in the metal container
below, a sort of enclosed dust shovel. He does his best to get as
much of the ash out of the oven as possible, but a tiny percentage
will, inevitably, stay lodged in the cracks of the brickwork. In the
metal container, the charcoal sits among the shards, glowing and
burning itself out until only the bones remain. Once cooled, the
bones go to the cremulator – a sort of blender with metal balls that
smash the bone into dust – and from there, to a plastic urn the
kind of colour you would expect to find ketchup in. Sometimes
it's green.

Every step of the way, a small printed card with the person's name on it is moved with them, from the cremator, to the metal container, to the bone blender, to the urn itself.

Not everything burns. Some bodily implants are removed before the body is laid in its coffin, lest they explode: in Poppy's mortuary in south London, after we had dressed Adam, I stood and watched as a short, bloodless slit was made in another dead man's chest and the pacemaker and its wires were pulled out from the place it held near his heart, while I, unconsciously, held the dead man's hand to comfort him. I didn't notice until the mortuary staff tried to wheel him away that I was, apparently, gripping him. He was a man with white hair unconstrained by gravity, like a flamboyant composer standing in a wind tunnel – a man generous enough to donate his body to science, whose gift was rejected for reasons we would never know. Instead, he was burned in a building like this, a little earlier than he had expected to be.

By the time bodies come to Tony, whatever implants are left inside are OK to go in the machine. He picks them out afterwards, when he's raking the bones, and places them in his bucket of battered metal joints and pins, which they used to bury in the cemetery but now have recycled. Other non-biological pieces – like the mercury in teeth – melt and escape into the atmosphere, or, in the case of breast implants that funeral directors sometimes forget to take out, stick like chewing gum to the bottom of the cremator.

Cancer is the last thing to burn. Tony doesn't quite understand why it happens; he thinks maybe it's the lack of fat cells, maybe the density of the mass – but when the rest of the body is gone, a tumour can sometimes remain, sitting black and still among the bones. Tony turns the gas jets on and shoot flames at it directly. The surface glows gold. 'It's almost like black coral,' he says.

Earlier that day, he had opened the furnace door to a cremation he describes now as 'nasty'. Whereas normally he might see a lump, this tumour appeared, to him, to be all through the body: from neck to pelvis. It was the body of a young woman whose photo was pinned to coffin wreaths that said 'DAUGHTER' and 'MUM', which will lie outside under a grapevine until a week from now, when Dave will put them in the bin.

'There's always something here that will get you,' says Tony, who seems choked up by this one cremation. 'That's why I struggle with the very religious. How can they believe in that when this is happening, and horrible bastards live to ninety? I'm not sure if there's a God looking down, but he's a funny geezer if there is.'

He keeps shaking his head imagining the pain she must have been in. He'd never seen anything like it in thirty years of manning these machines. (And neither has anyone else: I've asked a pathologist, an APT, an oncologist and an American crematorium worker, but nobody has seen this happen but Tony. It may be a quirk of the English machine, which runs at a lower temperature than American ones. The oncologist suggested maybe it was a calcification of the tissue. Mostly though, everyone was baffled.)

I remember the embalmer saying that when friends tell him about a cancer diagnosis, he extrapolates that information to its most extreme end point – death – and I wonder if hearing of a cancer diagnosis will now mean, to me, black coral in a crematorium. From the look on Tony's face, it's a hard image to forget. It feels like burying someone with the murder weapon, like something we should remove. Christopher Hitchens described the tumour in his oesophagus that would ultimately kill him as a 'blind, emotionless alien'. He later wrote, in his posthumously published book *Mortality*, that it was a mistake to ascribe animate qualities to inanimate phenomena. But I think there is no better way to describe a mass of flesh that will not burn, that will outlast its host – at least in an objective physical sense – if only for moments. Blind, emotionless, alien.

There's another funeral just finishing upstairs now. Tony's turned on the speakers so we can hear what's happening above piped down below: the calm of the funeral celebrant mixing with the growl of the machinery as it heats up: 850, 852. A beep sounds, and Betty Grey, in her MDF coffin with its plastic meltable handles, comes down on the lift.

The Hopeful Dead

Ripped and discarded tyres litter the scrubland. Among them, a microwave, a blown-out TV. An old antenna juts from the weeds by a collapsed chain-link fence. It's January, it's freezing, and the trees look like black bones against an overlit backdrop, a side-effect of the new LED streetlights distracting from the ruin around us by illuminating other things. Turn off a bright street where the restaurants and people are and the darkness is near total, like falling off the edge of the world, as if the game designer didn't reach this far. The car rolls to a stop and we look out at another abandoned house. The windows droop like tired eyes. Snow is beginning to fall on the banister to the second floor, roof yawning open to the electric glow of the sky.

Detroit is — or was, depending on how optimistic you are about its future — a city of dead American dreams. At its peak in 1950, it was the fourth most populated city in the country, the numbers lured here by a booming automobile industry and the promises that came with it. Since then, the city has been in decline, a diorama of America's rotten heart: deep-seated racism, corruption, the largest municipal bankruptcy filed in US history, the gulf between rich white people and everyone else — a striking city-wide example of the consequences of capitalism. The 1967 riots alone — by no means the first — left forty-three people dead, 7,231 arrested and 412 buildings destroyed. As the rich middle class bailed on the city, taxes went unpaid, ruins stayed ruins and time only added more: houses were burned in arson attacks the night before every Halloween. People continued to leave. The mayor tried to get those that stayed to move further in: they were living apart, in the last of the lone-standing houses on sprawling empty blocks.

Clint and I drive around in the dark, in another shitty rental car, looking for dinner, staring out at a John Carpenter set. A dirty black Dodge Challenger – an iconic car from the city's days as a formidable motor manufacturer – rumbles past us, over cracks in the road surface that look like an earthquake shook this postcode alone. We resolve that next time I convince him to drive me across America to interview somebody, I will rent a cooler car.

In 1995, Camilo José Vergara, a Chilean photographer who would take pictures of the same buildings year after year to chart their slow decay, had suggested that the city should be celebrated, that twelve blocks in downtown Detroit should be left to disintegrate, a monument to what happens if we let things die and decompose, if we allow other life to take over. The idea was met coldly by the people who still lived there – this was a living city in need of help, not a monument to death. Now, the MotorCity Casino Hotel rises high out of the dark, shooting multicoloured neon across its facade in green-red-purple-yellow streaks; a block away, homeless people warm themselves over a bin fire. Formerly grand skyscrapers turned spectacular ruins have been demolished to make way for car parks or empty lots. The bones of old office buildings have been cleared of birds and trees and turned into hotels. While it can, in places, feel like a city that is quietly resigned to its own dying, there is heartbreakingly conspicuous hope here.

In the early 1960s, there was a different kind of hope. Motown Records were all over the Billboard Charts and the label hadn't yet abandoned the place. Zoom out on the map and Neil Armstrong had not yet walked on the moon, but it was within reach. Zoom back in and a physics teacher called Robert Ettinger – then in his forties and increasingly aware of his own mortality, like anyone in their forties – wrote a book about how you could live forever. It was called *The Prospect of Immortality* and it made him, for a time, famous. He appeared on Johnny Carson's *Tonight Show* alongside Zsa Zsa Gabor.

The book wasn't a promise or a guarantee, it was exactly what it said on the cover: a prospect. It's a book about an idea – that death was a disease, and one not necessarily fatal – that began as a self-published pamphlet he believed might spark a movement if only he could get it into the right hands. His suggestion was to freeze a person at the moment of death and keep them from rot and decay until science caught up with whatever it was that killed them, reversing the damage to the point of life. The book is heavy on the science of freezing, light on how exactly the re-versal of death could happen, but that's the hope: that someone else will sort this out in the future, some greater minds in a more technologically evolved version of what we are now. The pace of scientific discovery was rapid – in Ettinger's own lifetime, human beings went from steam trains to space travel – and he had no reason to believe it would not continue at the same speed. He was not even the first to put forth the idea that death was not as per-manent as it seemed – religions, of course, have been doing that for millennia, and even Benjamin Franklin suggested something similar in 1773, wishing there was some way of embalming a dead person, maybe in a cask of Madeira, so that they might be revived a hundred years later to observe the state of America. But Ettinger was the first to take it so seriously and apply practical science to it outside of fiction. Fiction was, after all, where he had come across the idea originally, at twelve years old, in a short story by Neil R. Jones called *The Jameson Satellite*, published in 1931. In the story, a professor requests that after his death his body be fired into orbit, where it would be preserved indefinitely by the cold vacuum of space until it was awoken, millions of years later, by a race of mechanical men.

'Only those embrace death who are half dead already,' wrote Ettinger decades later, in the book that made him famous. 'The ones who surrender are those who are already in retreat.'

Ettinger is the reason I'm in Detroit. His frozen body hangs up-side down, bat-like, in a 'cryostat' tank inside a squat beige building a twenty-minute drive north of the unheated hotel room I froze in, horizontally, while a polar vortex blasted Michigan with arctic cold. In tanks alongside him hang his first wife, his second wife, and the first patient at the Cryonics Institute: his mother, Rhea.

§

Dennis Kowalski, president of the Cryonics Institute, is having a hard time trying to get his Skype to work. 'You don't need to see my ugly face anyhow,' he laughs. From their website I know he's about fifty, dark hair, a thick black moustache.

'I think it's kind of funny that you're hanging all your hope on technology reviving your corpse, but it's not even letting us do a video call without failing,' I say as I sit back, having given up on faffing around with settings.

'Well, I've always been an optimist,' says a voice from a screen that only has me on it.

I'm speaking to Dennis to find out what it's like to believe that death is not a permanent end, and why someone might devote this life to trying to get another one – it seems, to me, a waste of the first one. The cryonics people tend to get a bad rap in the press – they're painted as insane, delusional, a device for comedic farce: Fry from *Futurama* and Austin Powers were both awakened from their pods to futures they didn't understand, and Woody Allen's character in *Sleeper* was aghast to discover all of his friends had been dead for 200 years despite eating organic rice. (It's also because of these appearances in pop culture that 'cryogenics' gets confused with 'cryonics' – the former is a branch of physics that deals with the production and effects of very low temperatures, while it's only the latter that preserves corpses for later revival. The confusion annoys both parties.) Reading Ettinger's book, there's some nutty stuff in there – mostly about women and what to do with your multiple unfrozen wives – and by the end he has convinced himself so entirely that this is possible that he is certain that 'only a few eccentrics will insist on their right to rot'. But on the whole it seems optimistic and, above all, questioning. I wondered what kind of people in reality sign up to have their bodies frozen. When I called to find out, what I got, on the end of the line, was someone who seemed like a gentle nerd.

The Cryonics Institute has been running since 1976 and, at the time Dennis failed to get his Skype to work, had around 2,000 members, with 173 already frozen. He says there's no one 'type' of person who signs up, no one religion or political leaning, but if he had to pick a majority he'd say it was probably men, probably agnostic and probably Libertarian. They skew wealthier, but with the price tag of $28,000, which can be covered by life insurance (and is considerably lower than other cryonics companies, like Alcor in Arizona, at $200,000), they have poorer people too. This was important to Ettinger; in his book he said he didn't want his vision of the future to be so expensive that it would serve as a 'eugenic sieve'. I tell Dennis my theory that the transhumanist movement, into which cryonics tends to get lumped, seems to be mostly men because women watch their bodies start to fail earlier, in predictable stages, and that with their closer relation-ship to blood and birth, they're maybe more accepting of death and therefore less afraid – which might explain the numbers now weighted towards women working in the funeral industry. He's not so sure, but says maybe. He says it's not really about fearing death at all.

Young science-fiction fans, in my experience, tend to start out with a belief in a utopian future, and it's only later, when the real world creeps in, that dystopian ideas take root in the folds of their brains. With their toy rockets in their hands they think every-thing will be better one day because they have no reason yet to believe otherwise. It was around this utopian bubble period, in the mid-seventies, when Dennis was around seven or eight, that he caught an episode of *The Phil Donahue Show*. Bob Nelson, a former TV repairman, was on the show talking about the science of cry-onics and how he had, back in 1967, frozen the first man. Nelson had been a fan of Ettinger's book, and was a leader of one of the handful of cryonics groups that had sprung up around the country. The enthusiasts had taken Ettinger's theory and attempted to run with it.

The interview on *Donahue* wasn't enough to sell Dennis on cry-onics wholesale, and as spokesman for the movement Nelson didn't mention how wrong it was all going – how the bodies of his frozen clients were stored in a garage behind a mortuary, the coolant in their failing capsules topped up ever more infrequently as the money ran out and his own personal checks bounced, before the bodies were ultimately abandoned – but it sowed a seed.

'Then, when I was sixteen or seventeen, I would read *Omni* magazine, which took a lot of very deep science-fiction philosophy and brought it down to the layman's perspective,' says Dennis. 'They did an article about molecular nanotechnology and the reverse engineering of life. That was the blueprint.'

Dennis has been signed up at the Cryonics Institute for the last twenty years, and has been president of the organisation – a democratically run non-profit – for the last six. It's not his full-time job: outside of this, he's a paramedic in Milwaukee. 'I joke that in my day job I work in an ambulance saving lives, and in my night job I work in an ambulance to the future, *should that hospital exist*,' he says. 'It's the same thing in both ambulances: there's no guarantee that when you get in there we're going to save you.'

Before I spoke to Dennis, I had assumed he would be more convinced of the idea that he himself is now a spokesperson for. He keeps saying that nobody knows this will definitely work, but crucially nobody knows it definitely won't. 'Anyone that says cryonics is absolutely going to work is not a scientist. Anyone who says that it absolutely won't happen is not a scientist,' he says. 'The only way to find these things out is through the scientific method, which is running the experiment. We're basically all in a collective experiment in cryonics. Self-funded, no federal funding, no outside funding. Anyone else who is getting buried or burned is in the control group. Me, I'd rather be in the experimental group than the control group.'

He does, however, say there is anecdotal evidence to suggest that cryonics isn't as mad as it might look, that chances are leaning towards it actually working one day. He cites therapeutic hypothermia as something that is following the same line of reasoning as cryonics: lowering the temperature of the body (in this case after cardiac arrest) to slow things down and temporarily reduce the brain's need for nutrients and oxygen, because if those needs aren't met consciousness might never be regained. In *The Uninhabitable Earth: A Story of the Future*, David Wallace-Wells lists recently reanimated organisms: a 32,000-year-old bacterium in 2005, an 8-million-year-old bug in 2007, and in 2018, a worm that had been frozen in permafrost for 42,000 years. The *New York Times* reported that researchers had, in 2019, taken the brains out of the heads of thirty-two dead pigs and restored cellular activity to some of them. 'Stories seem to be coming out that are slowly but surely vindicating the logic of cryonics,' Dennis says. 'And if cryonics doesn't work, we're still advancing science by proving what's not possible. We're also helping out in other areas: we're dumping money into organ cryopreservation research because not only does it intrinsically benefit organ recipients, it also gets us one step closer to whole-body cryopreservation.'

Dennis says he doesn't want to prophesy and sell cryonics like it's some kind of religion, because that turns people off. He says the hardest thing is to get people to grasp the idea of being brought back from the dead – but we do that already, it just depends on what your definition of death is.

'A hundred years ago, when your heart stopped, you were done,' he says. 'You were dead. But today we routinely "bring people back to life". We shock them with defibrillators. We do CPR. We give them cardiac drugs. Sometimes those people walk out of the hospital, many times they don't. Electricity sounds like *Frankenstein*, but it's a big part of emergency medicine. Where would we be if we'd stuck with the notion that you can't ever bring people back to life?'

I always found the dystopian visions of the future more convincing in science fiction. Maybe it's all tied up in that one moment where I questioned the priest's story about God and the light bulb, perhaps my suspicion about an entity inhabiting machinery stretched to a general distrust of robots (and priests). To me, the brutal wasteland in Cormac McCarthy's *The Road* feels closer to a potential future reality, or the shining utopian facades that have rot under the surface, like ending lives at the ripe old age of thirty in *Logan's Run* (in the novel it was worse – you were finished at twenty-one). Any Philip K. Dick. To read the news and not despair at the projected graph of death and burning planetary destruction seems like a nice but alien idea to me. But Dennis never reached the dystopian phase; he is still planted wide-eyed and hopeful in the belief in a possible utopia, that there will be something worth coming back for – that not only is it possible he could live forever, but that the option is desirable.

'It might sound like I'm one of those people who can't face death, that I have to conjure up some sort of way out,' says the faceless voice from my speakers. 'But as a paramedic, I have seen people with do-not-resuscitate orders, and their family members are screaming at us to do something, to bring them back to a life of painful suffering when they didn't want to be brought back. That's the most extreme level of death denial. You need to understand death.'

§

The brain that hatched this plan of corpse reanimation remains inside Robert Ettinger's skull near the bottom of an insulated tank. The bodies are hung upside down because if there's ever a liquid nitrogen leak they want the most important part of you to be the last thing to thaw. It's likely they can grow you a new toe in the future, but probably not a brain – not the blueprint of who you are.

Outside of the building, Ettinger's neighbours include a door security system store, a lighting company headquarters, an auto repair shop and a heating induction service, all surrounded by neatly trimmed lawns and an occasional sad winter tree. A parked truck sits in the lot on its own, its side bearing the promise 'GREAT TIME PARTY RENTAL WE HAVE ALL OF YOUR PARTY NEEDS'. To get to the Cryonics Institute, you drive into this little cul-de-sac; you pass the party truck and follow the sign to the dead end.

I arrive at 10 a.m. on a snowy morning, Clint having driven through the manhole steam of Detroit to drop me off at the least space-age-looking building in town. A man in a big Midwestern puffer jacket waves his mitten at us through the glass door as we pull into the car park.

Before they moved here, the Cryonics Institute was closer to the city until they ran out of space. They don't plan on moving again; everyone that is here will stay here, they'll just buy up the buildings around them as the population grows. The frozen dead, slowly annexing the lighting company, the home security system head office, edging the party truck off the lot. This building is almost full, but there's one two doors down they've already bought, waiting to be set up for future cryonauts.

Hillary, twenty-seven, in her purple hoodie, jeans and Ugg boots, is going to take me on a tour of the facility. It's cold in here, but not freezing. It just feels like heating is not a thing they think about too much. Dennis mostly does his job remotely but says I'm in good hands: it's here that the three staff members deal with the practical business of storing the dead. Along with Hillary, there's Mike, the man with the mitten. He's Hillary's dad – she got him this job here, taking care of anything maintenance-related. Then there's Andy, shaved head with glasses, wearing a green sweatshirt, who quickly shakes my hand before getting back to work in the office at the front of the building with the window that looks out on the neat lawn. Most of the day-to-day jobs here, things like patient sign-ups and membership database entries, are a toss-up between Hillary and Andy; before she started here, Andy worked alone.

Hillary has shoulder-length brown hair and a delicate face; she's tiny, but for the last three years it has been she who deals most directly with the receiving and storing of the bodies. I drop my bag in the office and she takes me into a room not unlike the embalming room I saw in London, just emptier, tidier. Hillary herself is a trained embalmer, performing the 'perfusions' here, before the bodies are suspended in the tanks. (Perfusion is not a cryonics term: it broadly refers to the passage of blood – or a blood substitute – through the vessels or other natural channels in an organ or tissue. Chemotherapy drugs can be introduced to the body through perfusion. Embalming is perfusion. They just don't call it embalming here because what they're injecting is a different thing altogether.) There's a white porcelain table in the middle with a lip along the edge to stop fluids hitting the floor, space around it to manoeuvre bodies and gurneys, and endless cupboards of supplies all neatly tucked away. She moves to the corner and places her hand on the side of a tarpaulin bath resting on a gurney with half a CPR doll lying inside it, explaining that this is how the body of the recently dead is stabilised and transported to the facility: submerged in a portable ice bath, with blood circulation and breathing artificially restored by a heart-lung resuscitator. The machine keeps the blood circulating while the body is in the ice water, making it cool even faster by using the body's own machinery: its own pump, its own distribution service. They call it a 'thumper', like the rabbit. It looks like a toilet plunger suspended above a human chest. 'We've also got the mask, which gives them oxygen, so it keeps the blood oxygenated,' she says, pointing at the dummy's face. 'We try to keep as many cells alive as possible.'

If you die in America, you have to get to the Cryonics Institute within seventy-two hours if you want a perfusion – beyond that, your chances of a 'good' perfusion are lower – and many patients recorded on the website, where they publicly report the condition of every body, do not have a perfusion at all. To maximise your chances of making it in time, a company called Suspended Animation will (for a fee of between $60,000 and $102,000, depending on which services you select from the options menu) come and wait by your deathbed – any time wasted between death and ice will affect how well the next part of the process goes because any degeneration of the body will lessen the ability of the vascular system to distribute the solution. As soon as death is confirmed, they will place you in this bath, start the pump and bring you here. For less than $10,000 you can skip this bit, and rely solely on your local funeral director transporting your body to Hillary.

People who die in the UK have their perfusions done by embalmers trained by CI, before being shipped to the US for storage. (Kevin Sinclair, from the embalming room in London, is one of them. He said it was amazing to think that in several hundred years these people will be up and walking around again. When I asked him if he believed that to be true, he raised an eyebrow and said, 'No comment.') Pets, who are also frozen by CI if you'd like them to be – dogs, cats, birds, iguanas, whoever it is you want to bring with you to the future – generally get a better perfusion because the vet surgery is on the corner of this street. They go straight from being euthanised to here, arriving while they are still warm, when their blood hasn't been given a chance to settle or clot. It's for this reason that both Hillary and Dennis think euthanasia should be legalised for humans, but CI stays out of the conversation publicly, and at this point they do not accept any suicides, whatever the method – they don't want the possibility of another, better life to be the reason you ended this one.

By the sink are about sixteen bottles of clear liquid. Part of Hillary's job is to mix this liquid that takes the place of the salmon-pink embalming fluid. 'It prevents against freezing damage,' she says, picking up a bottle sort of apologetically, like she wished it was more interesting to look at. The way Dennis described the fluid, called CI-VM-1 (CI Vitrification Mixture One), to me over Skype, weeks ago, was that originally they would just 'straight-freeze' a person to liquid nitrogen temperatures and that was it – and they still do, to those people who missed the time window, or for whatever reason don't want this part of the process to happen. But they found that water freezing in the cells causes them to rupture, and the outside of the body freezing faster than the inside of the body causes interstitial damage – ice crystals forming in the spaces between things. So they hired a cryobiologist, who came up with a fluid that would allow them to freeze a body but leave its cells undamaged: a biological antifreeze that took its inspiration from the animal kingdom, from arctic frogs that freeze in the winter and come back in the spring, hearts beating, lungs breathing. In the frogs, as the temperature drops, special proteins in their blood suck the water out of the cells, while their liver pumps out huge amounts of glucose to prop up the cell walls. Humans don't have these proteins: when we freeze, we get frostbite and our cells collapse. This is what the liquid is trying to avoid. (For the straight-frozen patients, CI hopes that this is a problem the people in the future will have figured out. This is generally the answer to most questions.)

To inject the fluid into the body, they use a machine ordinarily used in open-heart surgery, mechanically reanimating the muscle so it performs its function as a pump and moves the chemicals around the vascular system. Hillary says it's a more accurate method than the traditional embalming machine I saw in London, simply because the pressure is easier to control – they keep the beat of the heart around 120 bpm, a moderate exercise level in a healthy adult, so that the liquid doesn't shoot through too fast and damage any of the vessels that are supposed to carry it. Though in principle it's a lot like embalming, the point of the fluid here is not to swell the bodies; it doesn't rehydrate the flesh or change the colour to make the person look alive, nor does it bloat them as they do in anatomy schools because they over-preserve them. Here, the fluid sucks the water out of the cells, dehydrating the whole body. Hillary says they look bronzed, sort of mummified. Shrunken. They take a grape and make a raisin.

The perfused body is then wheeled down the hall into the computer-controlled cooling room, where it lies in a cot at the bottom of what looks like a large chest freezer, wrapped in a shroud and insulating material similar to a sleeping bag, and strapped to a white backboard with ID tags attached – three per person. Over five and a half days it will be cooled slowly, in increments, to liquid nitrogen temperature – minus 196 degrees Celsius – the freezer spraying the body with liquid nitrogen whenever the computer tells it to. There is a laptop hooked up to it monitoring the process, and a battery backup in case the building loses power. Nothing that happens out here will affect the person cooling inside it. From there, they are lifted by the backboard out of the cooling tank via a system of ropes and chains attached to steel runners on the ceiling and lowered head first into one of the twenty-eight cryostats, the huge white cylinders that tower above us as we walk out of the perfusion room.

Hillary stops by a large rectangular container: a homemade-looking thing standing almost six feet tall with recesses in its outer walls like it was moulded in a waffle iron. White paint has dried in thick drips on the surface. She tells me that these were the first cryostats, made by hand out of fibreglass and resin by Andy, the man I met briefly in the office, who has been working here since 1985 and was there when they froze their first pa-tient. 'As you can imagine, it took a very long time to make, and they're expensive, so they switched to these cylinders,' she says, looking up at what she describes as a giant thermos bottle. These rely on no electricity to keep them cold, it all comes from within. Inside, holding up to six patients, there is a smaller cylinder, perlite insulation and a giant cork made of foam about two feet thick. Once a week, Hillary climbs the black steel ladder and spends four hours walking along the metal catwalk with a hose attached to pipes in the ceiling, topping up the level of the evaporating liquid nitrogen through a small hole in the lid of each tank.

We walk alongside them, each identical, no names anywhere. Hillary points at one of the cryostats where five small stones are lined up around the base. 'There is a dog of a Jewish family in there,' she says. 'Winston was his name, and he was their service dog. They live nearby and visit every couple of months.' It's a Jewish tradition to place a small stone by the grave every time you visit. A rabbi told me it's because, unlike flowers, stones do not fade. It's about the permanence of memory, of things lasting beyond their given time on earth.

It doesn't happen often, but people treat this place like a cemetery. Some bring stones, others bring birthday cards. You can visit as much as you like. You're just looking at a white tank with a logo instead of a headstone with a name. 'With funeral directing, you're with one person and then you move on. But with these people, we're here every day,' she says. 'We hear from the same family members that visit year after year. We're taking care of these people continuously.'

A couple of tanks down the line and on the left, Hillary stops and looks up at another white cylinder, as faceless and uniform as the rest. 'We have a young girl in here from the UK.' This girl made the news: she was only fourteen when she died, too young to make a will, and had written a letter to the High Court in England requesting that her body be frozen after her death – she knew she was dying of cancer, had discovered cryonics on the internet and wanted a chance of a cure in the future. Reporters climbed fences to try and get photographs of the facility, they rang the phones and the doorbell to try and speak to Hillary. She hid inside until they all went home.

Robert Ettinger, who died in 2011 at the age of ninety-two, is in the tank by the door of the boardroom. He was CI's 106th patient, his body put on ice within a minute of his last breath. Andy performed the perfusion. Despite the fact that it was his book that launched this whole thing, there is nothing to suggest he is here, and no mention of him anywhere on the walls bar one image. Ten feet away from where his body is stored, a black-and-white photo printed on canvas hangs at the head of the long boardroom table. He's wearing a suit and tie, he's a teacher smiling in front of a blackboard where algebraic equations are scrawled in chalk behind him. 'With a little bit of luck,' reads the quote on his photograph, 'we will taste the wine of centuries unborn.'

There is maths and science here, but it's not to dazzle, and none of it is certainty – all of it is a shrug and a maybe. There are no neon lights or promises of living forever on the walls – this meeting room looks no more technologically advanced than any other, they just have more inspirational quotes by Arthur C. Clarke. *Any sufficiently advanced technology is indistinguishable from magic.* The lights here are a little brighter, the indoor plants a little less funereal. There are no boxes of tissues placed on tables or on the arms of sofas. They've tried to make it a hopeful place.

This is the room where people come to ask any questions they want about the process before they sign up to have their bodies frozen. Hillary is the one who answers most of them. We sit and watch the memorial video, the pictures of some of the 155 pets in the building looping on the widescreen TV at the other end of the table. There goes Winston the service dog, a fluffy black poodle thing with ears that curl out like bunches. Angel, Thor, Misty, Shadow, Bunny, Rutgar. A black Labrador holds the screen just long enough for me to notice her red varnished nails. Then there's the people: old people, young people, Edgar W. Swank – president and last surviving founder of the American Cryonics Society, the oldest cryonics organisation still in existence – wearing the kind of glasses that only exist in science-fiction authors' photos. There are too many smiling young women who have died of incurable cancers. There's a lady from Hong Kong. Hillary remembers the ones she was there for, points them out as they flash by. 'She was young, I think she was in an accident. Linda, she was young too – cancer. He was recent – a heart attack.'

The Cryonics Institute's busiest year was 2018, with sixteen patients entering their cryostats. A lot of them were post-mortem sign-ups by their families, which Hillary thinks is probably down to the fact that word is spreading. Most of the new sign-ups are younger people – twenties, thirties. 'I think our age group sees a lot of potential with the technology,' she says. I ask if it's really about the trust in technology, or if it has something to do with the fear of death.

'Maybe a little of both,' she says. 'But I feel like, most of the time, it is more about just extending their life, and they see that possibility in the technology. People don't very often say that they're afraid of death and that's why they're doing this, but I do think it's part of it. I don't really think anybody wants to die.'

I assumed that someone who works here every day freezing the dead would have signed up to be one of them. But so far Hillary has not. 'It's not that I don't see the technology or believe in it, because I do. It's just a personal choice for me – I don't know if I want to come back,' she says, sounding not sad but pragmatic. 'I mean, life's hard. It's a struggle.' Her family aren't interested in cryonics, and she sees no point in coming back without them. She met her husband in mortuary school, and his family run six funeral homes in the area – she worked for them for a time, before she came here. Death has always been a certainty for him and he sees no need to change it. But I wondered when it became one for her.

'My mum got sick when I was fourteen,' she says. 'That was the wake-up call, because she had brain cancer and we knew she was going to die. I grew up very fast.' Two years later, her mother died, and because it had been a last request, her coffin lid was closed at the funeral; she didn't want people to see where part of her skull had been removed in surgeries, she didn't want them to see the weight gain from the steroids, she didn't want people to see her looking completely unlike herself. 'I understand her reasoning. But it bothered me,' says Hillary. 'I sat there looking at the coffin thinking, *Did they really put her in there? What did they do with her?*' It's Hillary's story, but it feels like I could have told it. In mine, I was twelve, and it was my friend in the coffin, but the scene is the same. How many people, especially children trying to understand, have, like us, sat in a church looking at a closed lid, thinking exactly the same things?

Something she misses now about funereal embalming is making a person look normal for their family again – she misses plumping up the withered shell of cancer patients, returning the colour to pallid cheeks. Because ultimately, all of this, for Hillary, is about caring for people. She had been the family of the sick person, she knew the strain and the anguish, and she learned from that experience what could be done better. She tried nursing school, but discovered sick people can be mean. She switched to mortuary school, worked in a funeral home, and liked everything about it except for speaking in front of the living – she's shy and quiet, and preferred being in the back room, on her own, with the body. And that's exactly what she does here.

She sounds apologetic again, like she should be more upbeat about the possibility of more life. 'I'm happy to be involved in this,' she says, the pictures of faces still flashing by on the screen at the end of the table. 'I feel like I'm doing something good. We don't know if it's for sure going to work, but I feel like I'm helping people get a chance.'

I'll be honest, I thought I was going to come here and find crazy people. I've spent so much time around those who work with death, who never question the finality of it, who work within the bounds of nature to make it less frightening than it feels, or show that it has worth. I thought I was going to meet people here who were certain of their ability to be revived, sure in their belief that it was also a good idea. I thought I would have to put on a reporter poker face, refrain from rolling my eyes at the idea that death was something that could be obliterated, that grief might be something you could avoid because the person wasn't really dead. But the people who visit this facility, who treat these cryostats as they would a grave, know grief all too well. For some, I'm sure, cryonics is the subconscious denial of death made conscious and ridiculous. But for others, this isn't the denial of death so much as humans allowing hope to glint in a night of despair. Hillary has thought about death to the point of zeroing in on the loneliness of eternal life – what is worth coming back for if everyone you love is gone? Then there is Dennis's qualified optimism, hedging his bets, preferring to be the experimental patient and not the control, while accepting none of this might work. There is more consideration here, more empathy than I expected to find in an institute founded on the belief that they could one day cheat the most fundamental fact of life. I came here to find out what it's like to live believing you won't die – that you won't ever meet the kind of death workers I have met – but that answer just isn't here.

Ultimately, I think, whether or not cryonics actually works may be a moot point. With climate change and the outlook for our continued existence on this planet looking bleak, there may never come a chance to find out. I personally don't think it will work, nor do I think it would be desirable if it did: Toni Morrison wrote that anything coming back to life hurts, and I believe her. Life is meaningful because it ends; we are brief blips on a long timeline colliding with other people, other unlikely collections of atoms and energy that somehow existed at the same time we did. Even in the best of circumstances, being reanimated could result in a permanent homesickness for a time and a place you cannot return to, a time and a place that no longer exist. But if none of this is hurting anybody – if it helps these people live, and if it helps them die – I see no reason to deprive them of their experiment, or to mock it. I like their optimism, but I do not share it. We do what we can to get by. It's a lullaby on a deathbed.

The next day, as my plane leaves Detroit Metro Airport, the same airport that receives the bodies destined for the cryostats, I look down at the snow and ice. Down there, somewhere, is the Cryonics Institute, where someone is on call at any hour of the day, any day of the year, ready to receive the hopeful dead. Maybe Hillary is walking the catwalk, filling up the tanks of people who hung those hopes on an ever-replenishing board of members who will advocate for them while they sleep, if they wake. From up here the snow brings out the footprints of the long-dead houses of Detroit like bark rubbings. The remaining houses stand frozen and alone, among the ghosts.

Afterword

It's late May, 2019. I've blown one deadline for this book and I'm about to miss another. I keep finding more people to speak to, more things I haven't thought about. I'm still thinking about the baby; I'm having a hard time concentrating on anything else. But right now, I'm in a bar overlooking Saundersfoot Bay in South Wales, interviewing a former detective sergeant, Anthony Mattick, about his work on murder cases. We're two pints in. I'm more tired than I've ever been in my life, the kind of exhaustion where sleep does nothing. I remember a line in David Simon's *Homicide*: 'Burnout is more than an occupational hazard in the homicide unit, it is a psychological certainty.' I figure Mattick is probably more tired than I am, but he doesn't seem to be.

He wears sunglasses on his head, tucked up on top of his short grey hair, but never puts them on. He's recently been in Spain for a joint fiftieth birthday party and is so sunburned he wouldn't look out of place on the executioner's plate at Red Lobster. Despite the view of the sunset over the sparkling sea, he's managing to clear the balcony by loudly telling me – in his baritone Welsh voice, between bursts of laughter – what he used to do for a living, back before an 18.5-tonne lorry picked him up off his bicycle and deposited him fifty yards down the road. He was airlifted to a hospital in Cardiff and died twice on the operating table. 'I got flattened. Smashed to bits!' he booms. 'My pelvis was blown open.' He's been retired for seven years, walking again for most of them. 'I was on an episode of *Ambulance*,' he adds, pissing himself laughing. Every sentence is 75 per cent words, 25 per cent cartoon facial explosion – whether he's talking about his own near-death experience or solving a murder case.

We leave the bar and its now-empty deck and walk through town trying to find somewhere that's still open for food at 9 p.m. It's a small coastal village; there's nowhere. Mattick waves at a bunch of teenage girls; they wave back. He shouts something cheery and unintelligible at a man spilling out of a pub; the man grins back. A cab driver greets him with 'Auto!' (Auto-Mattick, *geddit?*) and we pile into the car. I ask how he seems to know everyone in town. The teenage girls? He teaches at schools now, mentoring, that sort of thing. The guy outside the pub? Arrested him for burglary twenty years ago. 'You do your job right and there's no hard feelings,' he says, waving at someone else out the window.

Before his retirement, Mattick worked a range of cases over thirty years, all serious crime. He was part of the team that cracked the Pembrokeshire serial killer cold case, convicting John William Cooper, in 2011, of two double murders dating back to the 1980s. Mattick loved what he did, he loved being in the thick of it – so much so that he has signed up to be on call as part of Kenyon's disaster response team, having previously worked with Mo on plane crash victim recovery, picking up feet and heads on a mountain. 'I don't love it because of the … *macabreness,*' he says, his brow furrowing. 'There was a guy, a boss, lovely bloke, strong Carmarthen accent, he'd have a room full of detectives and he used to say – and he got this from someone who taught him, in the Met – *There's no greater privilege in life than being allowed to investigate the death of another human being.* That's a huge statement. It's massive. You are going to play a small part in doing that. Somebody is entrusting *you* to do that.'

We find the only restaurant in a nearby town that's still open – a Chinese, down a small backstreet – order most of the menu plus chips, and he tells me about the cases that stick in his mind. He's quieter now than he was on the balcony, digging up the stories while we wait for the spring rolls. But they're not buried all that deep.

Christmas Day, a dead baby. Three months old. Mattick left his own house on Christmas morning to visit the scene – a small property on the side of the road in the middle of nowhere. 'They were a lovely couple, had tried for the baby for years and years,' he says, looking pained. 'And you have to interview the parents, you have to get their statements. You have to make them feel comfortable, but you're still asking them the same questions as if they were guilty.' This is the side of the story I didn't see in the mortuary, as the police sat on their stools nearby, when Lara explained that SIDS is only ruled when everything else is ruled out. For Mattick, the smell of Christmas – the turkey, the tree, the cheap plastic and faint gunpowder of Christmas crackers – still brings it back to him: the wailing and the crying as he removed both the baby and the cot.

Another: a drowned father and son, fourteen days after they went missing, their bodies finally revealed by the low tide. The father's rigid hand still gripping a rock in the bay, the other holding the boy he had tried to save. 'Years later, I think: he died with his son. In his mind, he was thinking, I'm not letting go of my son. How could he, with two tides a day, and with the pull of the current, still hold onto a rock and hold onto his boy?' I nod, remembering Kevin the embalmer explaining that the physical manifestation of fear, like tension on a rollercoaster, can instantaneously freeze your muscles in place if that's the moment you die. It's called a cadaveric spasm. I wonder for a moment if Mattick is expecting more of a reaction out of me; I'm hearing the story of a dead father and son and thinking about the practical cause of the grip, the chemicals in the body. How would I have reacted before I started this book? I imagine I would have asked about the mother. But I don't.

He empties the rest of the bottle of wine into my glass and signals for another one, finding a place for it on the last patch of table not covered by plates and spilled fried rice. Then he goes on, recalling a man on fire on CCTV. 'Most of the people I see are dead, but this was somebody *dying*,' he says. 'I've seen knives, guns, heads blown off, mouths blown off. An elderly man who was just the outer shell, the rest of him had dripped through the ceiling because he had been left so long. Wash-ups on the beach. One where a train chopped a guy in half – I had the legs, my mate had the other half. I've seen a girl, ejected out the back of a car – the whole back of her skull was missing. The nurse was doing mouth-to-mouth at three in the morning, on the road, and as she blew in her mouth she was spraying gunk all over my feet. The girl had no brain, nothing left, it had all fallen out. The nurse didn't know, she couldn't see the level of trauma – she had no light. She was blowing, but it didn't sound right. It was coming right out the back of her head. I said to her, "I'm so sorry." She looked up, she had blood round her face.'

He shovels some more food onto his plate while I sit with the image of a nurse on her knees, trying desperately in the dark. He's already moved on to the next story, chuckling now. 'Another one, a guy, he was huge. Died upstairs, we couldn't get him down the beautiful wooden staircase. The undertaker had to cough to mask the sound of us snapping him in half to get him round the bend,' he's laughing into his napkin.

'The sound of rigor snapping is pretty memorable,' I say, because what else do you say after a list like that, though I realise later, while listening to the interview tape, that 'Oh my God' or 'Fuck' might have been more normal.

'You've heard it?' Mattick says, eyebrows raised behind his napkin. He puts it back down on his lap and looks at me like he's not sure what we're here for any more. I'm supposed to be the one who hasn't seen anything, the one asking what it's like. So I tell him what I've been doing. I tell him about the bodies in the mortuaries, the skull in the ash, the coffin on the hill. I tell him about the brain in my hands and the baby in the bathtub. I notice I'm listing them like he did.

'You're asking me about stuff that you're already going through,' he says. 'I'm not taking the piss. You're asking me what sticks with me, and you've already got things in you. I don't mean to turn it on you, but that's what it is. I'm surprised you haven't gone through six bottles on your own! And you're asking *me* questions? You're already there, mate. You have, um, *gone for it.*'

I shrug awkwardly, my face saying what I hope comes across as, *I didn't mean to, not this much.* In the beginning, the plan was simple: I was going to interview death workers about how they do their jobs and how they deal with it all in their heads; maybe they'd show me if I kept out of the way. I was going to follow the body from mortuary to burial and report on what I saw. I've interviewed hundreds of people before, about lots of different things: films, boxing, typefaces, stories both happy and sad. I'm a tourist in various worlds, and I figured I would be a tourist in this one, packing up my notepad and voice recorder and leaving when I was finished – I don't think you can see something once and call yourself a local, no matter how much you pay attention. Even so, I had seen more than I expected to. I had felt more than I expected to. 'Honestly, I was fine with everything except for the baby,' I tell him, because it's true. I was busy looking at the avalanche and it was the small bouncing pebble that got me right between the eyes.

Maybe Mattick is right. Maybe I've seen enough – I'm 'already there'. Maybe this is my last interview; he's just given me the green light to stop.

Neither of us says anything. Mattick has stopped eating. He's looking at me, mentally updating where he thinks I'm at. Earlier, at the bar, it had taken some encouragement to get him to talk openly about his work – he was giving me the headlines (loudly), the pre-watershed broadcast. He assumed I hadn't seen any of it, and that I didn't *actually* want to hear the details because experience has taught him that no one ever does, not really, and the dispersing crowd at the bar didn't convince him otherwise. It was hours before he told me about the nurse on her knees and the old man dripping through the ceiling. I've made no assumptions with you, reader, about what you can handle – it would be antithetical to what I was trying to do, conceding to the cultural barriers I was trying to go beyond – and now you're here with me. The sound of the restaurant fills the silence between me and Mattick.

'The thing is, now...' He sits back and stares off to the corner of the room, past the golden cat with the waving hand, deciding whether or not to say whatever it is he's about to say. 'No, I'll come out with it because you're doing the book – don't take it the wrong way.' He leans forward, serious. '*You'll never get rid of the pictures.* I don't mean that to be nasty. There will be triggers that will bring these things back to you. You'll be somewhere, and you won't know why, but all of a sudden it will crop up. And you won't be able to stop it. Because what you've seen isn't normal. The things you were asking me about – you've just stepped into it.'

He tells me that it's down to where and how I file away the images: that right now they're at the forefront, but soon they won't be. 'I've been doing this thirty years,' he says. 'Nurses do it. Firefighters do it. You're going to have to be able to detach yourself, or you're going to wonder what the hell you were doing.'

It makes perfect sense to me now, all those times the people I've spoken to have said they talk to their colleagues, rather than a therapist, when something has got to them – someone who was there, who saw what they saw – whether it's Clare and her fellow midwives in the break room or Mo at an annual barbecue. Funeral directors, embalmers and APTs trade stories at conferences, knowing that no one around them will flinch. Many of them remind me of what I've read about soldiers who feel they can only talk to other soldiers because their frames of reference are so out of the ordinary, the context so far removed from everyday life. They want someone with a shared experience, not just a clinical understanding. I don't have colleagues who understand. So I sit at a computer and I type it all up. I tell Mattick that the baby is so much on my mind that I sit beside people in cafes with their babies in their baskets and I picture them dead. Or my friends casually mention they sleep with their baby between them and statistics on co-sleeping deaths flash in my mind. I tell him I'm no fun at parties because I will corner someone and tell them about the baby. It doesn't take much. All they have to do is ask me how I am.

'But I'll be amazed if you say it hasn't made you more appreciative,' he says. 'It will change you, in a nice way. A lot of the time it makes you very humbled. You look at the babies, and even though your mind's going one way, you appreciate it more – you've seen the other side. To me, the expression is it makes you *better*. I don't mean better than somebody else, what I mean is it makes you better in yourself. You will be able to see things better. Do things better. Because you've been exposed to things that generally people aren't going anywhere near. And rightly so.' I nod. If nothing else, my time being around the dead has made me more patient with people, which might explain why so many death workers have been so patient with me, so open with someone they had only just met. I argue less. I still get angry, but it feels muted. As a champion grudge-holder, I have now forgotten most of them.

'Do you have any regrets about putting yourself in the position you did with your job?'

'That's one word that doesn't feature,' he says, completely certain of it. 'I've never, ever regretted. I can be corny now and say we're all on a journey – you've chosen yours. You make a decision, you go with it. The worst thing you can do is not finish it. Then you'd have a regret.'

§

In psychiatrist Bessel van der Kolk's book *The Body Keeps the Score*, about the clinical basis of trauma in the mind and body, he writes that the body responds to extreme experiences by secreting stress hormones, which are often blamed for subsequent illness and disease. 'However, stress hormones are meant to give us the strength and endurance to respond to extraordinary conditions. People who actively *do* something to deal with a disaster – rescuing loved ones or strangers, transporting people to a hospital, being part of a medical team, pitching tents or cooking meals – utilise their stress hormones for their proper purpose and therefore are at much lower risk of becoming traumatised.' These death workers, these 'helpers' as Fred Rogers might say, can deal with it mentally because they are dealing with it physically – they are *doing* something while we (while I) sit by. 'Nonetheless,' van der Kolk continues, 'everyone has his or her breaking point, and even the best-prepared person may become overwhelmed by the magnitude of the challenge.'

The thing I discovered again and again in speaking to people who work with the dead is that nobody takes it in all at once. Nobody sees the whole of death, even if death is their job. The death machine works because each cog focuses on their one patch, their corner, their beat, like the worker in the doll factory who paints the face and sends the doll off somewhere else for her hair. Nobody collects the dead body from the roadside, autopsies it, embalms it, dresses it and pushes it into the fire. It is a series of people, connected in their industry, disconnected in their roles. There is no prescribed antidote to the fear of death, but your ability to function within its realm depends on where you look, and as crucially, where you don't. I have met funeral directors who tell me they could not handle the gore of an autopsy, a crematorium worker who could not dress a dead man because it is too personal, and a gravedigger who can stand neck-deep in his own grave in the day but is scared of the cemetery at night. I have met APTs in the autopsy room who can weigh a human heart but will not read the suicide note in the coroner's report. We all have our blinkers on, but what we block out is personal to us.

All of these death workers have their limits, but each of them is considered – they are there so nobody becomes overwhelmed by the magnitude of the challenge. When Mattick talks about detachment, I believe it's a constructive detachment rather than a cold one: putting the scene in context, allowing himself space in order to perform his job effectively without collapsing. He wants me not to bury the things I have seen, not to ignore them and block them out, but to put them in a context that is meaningful. It's a different kind of detachment from the type I saw in the executioner, who had rewritten his reality to a point where he was barely part of it, who in this new narrative had denied himself any sense of agency as a way of making peace with what he had done. Or the crime scene cleaner, who doesn't want to know the story, who deliberately removes the image from its context so all that remains is the blood – and a countdown clock on his phone until the day he can detach himself for good.

If there is anything I want you to take from this, it's that you should consider where your own limits might be. Throughout this entire experience, I was seeing limits put in place by other people: the father of the stillborn baby making it disappear while the mother slept; the unviewable Vietnam soldier returned in a coffin with the metal lid bolted down; the man coming to Poppy in her funeral home, asking if she would let him see his drowned brother because no one else would. These limits are often arbitrary, institutionalised assumptions that do nothing for us. I believe that limits should be personal to you, chosen by you, and as long as you have carefully considered them rather than allowed them to be dictated by cultural norms, they are right. 'We're not here to force a transformational experience on people who don't want it,' Poppy said to me, sitting in her wicker chair way back at the start of everything. 'Our role is to prepare them, to gently give them the information they need in order to make an empowered decision.' I believe she is right. The world is full of people telling you how to feel about death and dead bodies, and I don't want to be one of them – I don't want to tell you how to feel about anything, I only want you to think about it. Some of the richest, most meaningful and transformative moments of your life may lie beyond where you think your limits currently are. Help dress your dead if you feel you are able, or even if you're just curious. We are stronger than we give ourselves credit for. Ron Troyer, the retired funeral director, learned this long ago, when he pried that lid off the soldier's coffin, when the father looked at his son returned from the war; he did not see horror, he saw his boy.

I have thought, often, of a woman I met years ago, who told me about her mother dying in hospital. She didn't go to see her because she didn't want her final image to be one of death, so she let her mother die alone. She was sixty and had never seen a dead body before, and she imagined that a lifetime of memories could be replaced by a single one in a hospital bed. She believed that it was the image of death that would irreparably break something inside her, rather than the fact of her loss. I think there is urgent, life-changing knowledge to be gained from becoming familiar with death, and from not letting your limits be guided by a fear of unknown things: the knowledge that you can stand to be near it, so that when the time comes you will not let someone you love die alone.

As for my own limits, there were times when I wished I hadn't seen the baby. But without that moment there would be a whole world of human grief and experience that would remain invisible to me. I would never have met Clare, the bereavement midwife, and it was her job more than any other that highlighted how underappreciated so many of these people are, how little we know about them, and how much they contribute not just to the management of our dead, but the management of our minds and hearts. Those who live through a traumatic experience shouldn't be the sole keepers of that knowledge; it is because of the work of people like Clare – who not only takes the photographs for the memory boxes but remembers them herself, and sees this validation of existence as a crucial part of her job – that such experiences become less alienating, less isolating. Where does empathy come from if not seeing and trying to understand?

Trying to understand something invisible was, after all, the basis for this whole endeavour, and for me to reject one part of it would undermine my intention. I wanted to see all of it. But in many of these rooms, standing in front of these bodies, I was, for a few moments, speechless. As a journalist I'm usually full of questions, but there are parts of interview tapes where I have none – there's dead air, the hum of a freezer, the sound of a bone saw. I would get home and I'd be mad at myself for occasionally faltering, for not looking at the photograph on Adam's chest, or for not stepping closer when the decapitated cadaver was casually unveiled by a student who had no idea why I was there. I'd exchanged a hundred pleading emails and travelled thousands of miles to get close to the dead, why not a few more feet to examine the neatness of the cut Terry had made? What stopped me in that moment? A sense that this was not my place, that even though I was standing in the room I could still only watch from a distance? Or did I think, back then, that I couldn't handle seeing the stump of a spine? I was standing, reacting and trying to do my job at the exact intersection of wonder and fear: 'The two incommensurate human emotions strike and collide,' wrote Richard Powers, 'throwing off sparks that might equally burn or warm.'

Sometimes, when it got hard, I would ask myself what it was, exactly, that I was looking for. After seeing the first dead body in

Poppy's mortuary, had I not seen real death as I had wanted to all those years ago? What else was there to find?

In the days after I spoke to Mattick, I couldn't shake the image of the dead father holding his son while clinging to the rock in the bay. It had a grip on my heart that I couldn't articulate, that I couldn't get straight in my mind. When he told me about them that night in the Chinese restaurant, I took the facts of the scene and explained them to myself with what I now knew of biological functions in death. It was reductive, detached in the same way the crime scene cleaner is detached. I wasn't seeing the whole picture. It nagged at me for weeks, until finally I saw what was revealed by the receding tide.

The muscles cannot freeze what isn't there. A cadaveric spasm is not regular rigor mortis, it's a rare form of muscle stiffening that is stronger than rigor – it cannot be undone as easily as I watched Sophie in the embalming room bend the knees of the man in front of her. A cadaveric spasm happens at a moment of extreme physical tension, a moment of intense emotion. The people who found the father and his son had time-travelled to their final moment, a still life under the waves. The low tide uncovered what death had preserved: the father's final impulse to never let go of his son. The currents in the bay are strong, and nobody drowns instantly – had this impulse been weaker, his fingers would have slipped away from the rock, their bodies would have been found elsewhere and apart. It was the same primal impulse I felt standing next to the baby in the mortuary as he went under the water – I wanted to reach out and grab him, and if it meant I could save his life, I would never let go.

Now I see all of it: death shows us what is buried in the living. By shielding ourselves from what happens past the moment of death we deny ourselves a deeper understanding of who we truly are. 'Show me the manner in which a nation cares for its dead and I will measure with mathematical exactness, the tender mercy of its people, their respect for the law of the land and their loyalty to high ideals,' goes the William Gladstone quote, framed on the wall of Mo's office at Kenyon. We are cheating ourselves out of knowing this, with our system of payments and disappearances. These unseen acts of care, the tender mercies of these death workers, show not a cold detachment from their work, but the opposite – some kind of love.

In the brief time I've been around death I think I've become more tender, yet also more toughened: accepting how all of this ends, I find myself mourning people while they're still here. I have a collection of photos of the back of my father's silver head as he leans over his drawing board, the pictures of the five dead women now long gone. Images on a laptop – all I had in a time when we were geographically separated by a pandemic, by a world shut down, when dying alone became the fate of thousands. This book became a personal reckoning with the trickle, shortly before the flood.

§

In January 2020, during the early days of the coronavirus pandemic, a single image of a dead Chinese man flat on his back in the street was, to me, the most telling evidence we had of the approaching cataclysm. There he lay, with his medical mask on his face. The reporters said that in the two hours they observed the scene, at least fifteen ambulances drove past on their way to other calls before a blacked-out van arrived to zip him into a body bag and disinfect the pavement where he'd been. At that point, the virus was still a distant fate, something happening to someone else. But it only takes one body out of place to signal the breakdown of something fundamental. If the bodies were staying where they fell, the death workers were struggling to cope. They work on part of the frontline that nobody claps for. Theirs is a job most noticeable in absence.

After that Chinese man, images of actual death were harder to come by in the UK press, while the government played down the threat of what was coming. As the death toll mounted, media focused more on the stories of support for the NHS, or on Captain Tom, a ninety-nine-year-old former British army officer raising money by walking slow lengths of his garden. But if deaths are just numbers on a screen every day, the reality of an invisible enemy is easier to trivialise. Down in the mortuary, an overworked Lara swapped her paper surgical mask for a rubber respirator; elsewhere, people debated the existence of the virus. News outlets tried to show us, eventually, what the inside of hospitals looked like, but unless you searched for the stories, you didn't see coffins or body bags or temporary mortuaries – if you did, they were usually in a different country. 'The more remote or exotic the place, the more likely we are to have full frontal views of the dead and dying,' wrote Sontag, in her book about our response to images of pain.

At the time it felt, to me, like we were missing a huge piece of the story, but also that this failure to understand began long before the events of 2020. How can you translate digits into dead bodies, when death is already treated as abstract?

It reminded me of something the AIDS activist Cleve Jones had said to Terry Gross on an episode of *Fresh Air*, years ago. He was talking about being in San Francisco in 1985, when the AIDS death toll of the city had just reached 1,000. That November, he was at the annual candlelight tribute to the assassinated politicians Harvey Milk and George Moscone, standing on the corner of Castro and Market, when he became overcome with frustration at the lack of visible evidence: here he was in the epicentre of an epidemic that was rapidly spreading, yet was barely acknowledged outside of the community. All around him people were sitting in restaurants, laughing, playing music. He said, 'I thought to myself, if we could knock down these buildings, if this was a meadow with a thousand corpses rotting in the sun, then people would look at it and they'd understand it. And if they were human beings, they would be compelled to respond.' Instead of destroying, he began creating: he started the AIDS Memorial Quilt, each piece six feet by three feet, the approximate size of a grave. Thirty-six years later, it still grows: names honoured on the quilt number 105,000. It weighs fifty-four tons. It's the largest piece of community folk art in the world. And it is there because the bodies are hard to conceive of, and easy to ignore, if you cannot see them – or your prejudice says they don't matter.

In 2020, people were saying breathless goodbyes on small screens. Some were seeing death for the first time, and it was someone they loved. We were unable to mourn in the usual ways: we couldn't attend their funerals, but many were broadcast on Zoom – another thing on another screen. We were left with just the *idea* of death. In April, when the world had trouble sleeping, BBC Radio 3 teamed up with the European Broadcasting Union to simulcast Max Richter's *Sleep*, an eight-hour lullaby, across fifteen channels in Europe, the USA, Canada and New Zealand.

Action rarely looks like inaction, but in this crisis you could save lives by sitting on your sofa, staring at the wall. The psychological impact of lockdown was not just that we were inside, alone, or crowded in with our families: we had all of these stress hormones and nothing to do with them. Inertia bred anxiety and a feeling of hopelessness – never knowing the quantifiable effect of what your doing nothing did. Over 250,000 people in the UK volunteered to be a helper to have some tangible hold on the world as it fell apart.

As the daily death toll crept from the single digits to the forties, doubling every few days until it hit the hundreds and thousands, I thought: each of these is a person, a body in a bag. Someone, somewhere, took care of every one of them, just like someone did with my friend when they pulled her from that flooded creek. Some of them are in this book that I started long ago, and finished in a city locked down. Stuck in the house – my brain turned to mush by stress and uselessness – I noticed for the first time, like a lot of people, the garden. I hadn't previously cared beyond standing at the back door throwing scraps of dinner to the family of crows we had befriended. But I started, very tentatively, to cut down the vines and brambles that had swallowed small trees. I took pictures of other things to figure out if they were supposed to be there or if they too were a weed. After weeks of hacking, pulling and digging in the kind of clay that makes a perfect burial plot but a difficult garden, I started to plant things. I watched tiny life sprout from the soil no matter what happened in the news, no matter how little I knew, no matter how many people died. The relent-lessness of nature was emotionally sustaining, but none of this was a distraction from what was happening beyond the garden gate: it was a way of processing it.

Thinking about death and the passage of time is part of tending a garden. You put things in the ground knowing they might fail. You grow things knowing they will die with the frosts six months from now. An acceptance of an end and a celebration of a short, beautiful life is all tucked up in this one act. People say gardening is therapeutic, that putting your hands in soil and effecting change on the world makes you feel alive and present, like something you do matters even if it's only in this one terracotta pot. But the therapy runs deeper than physicality: from the start of spring, every month is a countdown to an end. Every year, the gardener accepts, plans for and even celebrates death in the crisping seed heads that sparkle with ice in winter: a visible reminder of both an end and a beginning.

As the cold came, so did more death. In New York, freezer trucks that had been parked outside hospitals for extra mortuary space in the first wave were still there: 650 bodies on the Brooklyn waterfront belonging to families who either could not be located or could not afford a burial. Los Angeles county temporarily suspended air-quality regulations and lifted the limit on monthly cremations to tackle the backlog. In Brazil, when the daily death toll spilled over 4,000, nurses on Covid isolation wards filled nitrile gloves with warm water and placed them in the hands of patients to simulate human touch, so they wouldn't feel alone. Back in late March 2020, standing in the Rose Garden – hundreds of thousands of deaths ago – President Donald Trump said, 'I wish we could have our old life back. We had the greatest economy that we've ever had, and we didn't have death.'

We've always had death. We've just avoided its gaze. We hide it so we can forget it, so we can go on believing it won't happen to us. But during the pandemic, death felt closer and possible, and everywhere – to everyone. We are the survivors of an era defined by death. We will have to move the furniture of our minds to accommodate this newly visible guest.

Notes

I have put quote marks around direct quotes from the source, otherwise they are references.

EPIGRAPH

'Life is tragic simply because the earth turns': James Baldwin, *The Fire Next Time*, Penguin, 2017 edition, p. 79.

INTRODUCTION

my dad – Eddie Campbell, a comic book artist – was working on a graphic novel: Alan Moore and Eddie Campbell, *From Hell*, Top Shelf Productions, San Diego, 1989, 1999.

On average, 6,324 people in the world die every hour – that's 151,776 every day, about 55.4 million a year: World Health Organisation, 'The Top 10 Causes of Death', 9 December 2020. <who.int/news-room/fact-sheets/detail/the-top-10-causes-of-death>

Becker considered death to be both the ender and the propeller of the world: Ernest Becker, *The Denial of Death*, The Free Press, New York, 1973.

'How can you be sure it is death you fear?': Don DeLillo, *White Noise*, Penguin, New York, 2009, p. 187. Reproduced with permission of Pan Macmillan, the Licensor, through PLSclear (UK). Also with permission of Penguin Random House LLC (US).

THE EDGE OF MORTALITY

a shy academic in charge of Bentham's care had shown it to me for a piece I was writing: Hayley Campbell, 'This Guy Had

Himself Dissected by His Friends and His Skeleton Put on Public Display', BuzzFeed, 8 June 2015. <buzzfeed.com/hayleycampbell/why-would-you-put-underpants-on-a-skeleton>

I remember the filmmaker David Lynch, in an interview, talking about visiting a mortuary: David Lynch: The Art Life, dir. Jon Nguyen, Duck Diver Films, 2016, DVD, Thunderbird Releasing.

Denis Johnson wrote about this smell … ethyl mercaptan, the first in a series of compounds brought out in the process of putrefaction: Denis Johnson, The Largesse of the Sea Maiden, Jonathan Cape, London, 2018, in the short story Triumph Over the Grave, p. 121.

'The edge of death and dying is around everything like a warm halo of light': David Wojnarowicz, Close to the Knives, Canongate, Edinburgh, 2017, p. 119. © David Wojnarowicz, 1991. Extracts from Close to the Knives: A Memoir of Disintegration reproduced with permission of Canongate Books Ltd (UK) and Vintage/Penguin Random House LLC (US).

THE GIFT

In 1883, three decades after the town was founded, a tornado tore the place apart: Ken Burns Presents: The Mayo Clinic, Faith, Hope, Science, dir. Erik Ewers and Christopher Loren Ewers, 2018, DVD, PBS Distribution.

'You know this shit is bad when you gotta go to the fucking North Pole to find out what's wrong with you': Billy Frolick, 'Back in the Ring: Multiple Sclerosis Seemingly Had Richard Pryor Down for the Count, but a Return to His Roots Has Revitalized the Giant of Stand-Up', LA Times, 25 October 1992. <latimes.com/archives/la-xpm-1992-10-25-ca-1089-story.html>

a WIRED magazine article about a new, more environmentally sound method of cremating bodies with super-heated water and lye instead of fire: Hayley Campbell, 'In the Future, Your Body Won't Be Buried … You'll Dissolve', WIRED, 15 August 2017. <wired.co.uk/article/alkaline-hydrolysis-biocremation-resomation-water-cremation-dissolving-bodies>

The shift from carrying out dissections on animals to the human dead was a focus of political, societal and religious tension: All historical facts on body donation rely heavily on Ruth Richardson, Death, Dissection and the Destitute, Penguin, London, 1988, pp. xiii, 31–2, 36, 39, 52, 54, 55, 57, 60, 64, 260.

When I saw it in an exhibition in 2012, it was placed on the same shelf as a slice of Einstein's brain: Marius Kwint and Richard Wingate, Brains: The Mind as Matter, Wellcome Collection, London, 2012.

'This my will and special request I make, not out of affectation of singularity': Jeremy Bentham, quoted by Timothy L. S. Sprigge, The Correspondence of Jeremy Bentham, vol. 1: 1752 to 1776, UCL Press, London, 2017, p. 136.

since the rise in bequests coincides with an increased cremation rate, perhaps the spiritual associations of the corpse had changed in the post-war period: Richardson, Death, Dissection and the Destitute, p. 260.

Today's UK medical cadavers are now exclusively the bodies of those who have donated them, which isn't true of everywhere in the world: Figures found in a study by Juri L. Habicht, Claudia Kiessling, MD and Andreas Winkelmann, MD, 'Bodies for Anatomy Education in Medical Schools: An Overview of the Sources of Cadavers Worldwide', Academic Medicine, vol. 93, no. 9, September 2018, Table 2, pp. 1296–7. <ncbi.nlm.nih.gov/pmc/articles/PMC6112846>

'Anatomy is the very basis of surgery … it informs the head, gives dexterity to the hand, and familiarises the heart with a sort of necessary inhumanity': William Hunter, 'Introductory Lecture to Students', St Thomas's Hospital, London, printed by order of the trustees, for J. Johnson, No. 72, St. Paul's Church-Yard, 1784, p. 67. Provided by Special Collections of the University of Bristol Library. <wellcomecollection.org/works/p5dgaw3p>

Wyoming – a state in the heart of the American male suicide epidemic: 'Suicide Mortality by State', Centers for Disease Control and Prevention. <cdc.gov/nchs/pressroom/sosmap/suicide-mortality/suicide.htm>

Calen Ross shot himself and died in south-western Minnesota: Associated Press, 'Widow Gets "Closure" after Meeting the Man Who Received Her Husband's Face', USA Today, 13 November 2017. <eu.usatoday.com/story/news/2017/11/13/widow-says-she-got-closure-after-meeting-man-who-got-her-husbanmtouches-man-who-got-her-husbands-fac/857537001>

To prepare for the operation, the surgeons, nurses, surgical technicians and anaesthetists spent fifty weekends in Terry's lab: 'Two Years after Face Transplant, Andy's Smile Shows His Progress', Mayo Clinic News Network, 28 February 2019. <newsnetwork.

mayoclinic.org/discussion/2-years-after-face-transplant-andy-sandness-smile-shows-his-progress>

CLICK YOUR FINGERS AND THEY TURN TO STONE

Published (in English) in 1929, it's a collection of death masks ranging from the fourteenth century up to the twentieth: Ernst Benkard, *Undying Faces*, Hogarth Press, London, 1929.

Kate O'Toole laughed that it was 'classic O'Toolery' that he would end up in the mortuary drawer beside Biggs: *Death Masks: The Undying Face*, BBC Radio 4, 14 September 2017. Produced by Helen Lee. <bbc.co.uk/programmes/b0939wgs>

The British Conservative politician Jacob Rees-Mogg had his father's face cast: Ibid.

You can see Nick's process for making a death mask in a grainy three-minute video on YouTube: *Amador*, Resistor Films, YouTube, 9 November 2009. <youtu.be/zxb9dMYdmx4>

at UCL are thirty-seven masks they don't know what to do with, remnants of a long-dead phrenologist's collection: Hayley Campbell, '13 Gruesome, Weird, and Heartbreaking Victorian Death Masks', BuzzFeed, 13 July 2015. <buzzfeed.com/hayleycampbell/death-masks-and-skull-amnesty>

'The Thief of the Century': Duncan Campbell, 'Crime', *Guardian*, 6 March 1999. <theguardian.com/lifeandstyle/1999/mar/06/weekend.duncancampbell>

'no live organism can continue for long to exist sanely under conditions of absolute reality': Shirley Jackson, *The Haunting of Hill House*, Penguin, New York, 2006, p. 1. Reproduced with permission of Penguin Random House LLC (US).

LIMBO

According to Richard Shepherd, the forensic pathologist in charge of London and south-east England at the time, it was one of a series of disasters that revolutionised things: Richard Shepherd, 'How to Identify a Body: The *Marchioness* Disaster and My Life in Forensic Pathology', *Guardian*, 18 April 2019. <theguardian.com/science/2019/apr/18/how-to-identify-a-body-the-marchioness-disaster-and-my-life-in-forensic-pathology>

it's a common occurrence for close relatives to have doubts about, deny or mistakenly agree to the identity of a deceased person: *Public Inquiry into the Identification of Victims following Major Transport Accidents*, Report of Lord Justice Clarke, vol. 1, p. 90, quoting Bernard Knight, *Forensic Pathology* (2nd edition, chapter 3), printed in the UK for The Stationery Office Limited on behalf of the Controller of Her Majesty's Stationery Office, February 2001.

'However ... that person clearly did not know that not seeing them is even worse': Richard Shepherd, *Unnatural Causes: The Life and Many Deaths of Britain's Top Forensic Pathologist*, Michael Joseph, London, 2018, p. 259. Reprinted by permission of Penguin Books Ltd. (UK), © 2018 Richard Shepherd.

In March 1991, United Airlines Flight 585, a Boeing 737-200, was approaching Colorado Springs to land: National Civil Aviation Review Commission, Testimony of Gail Dunham, 8 October 1997. <library.unt.edu/gpo/NCARC/safetestimony/dunham.htm>

it rolled to the right, pitched nose-down until near vertical and hit the ground: 'United Airlines – Boeing B737-200 (N999UA) flight UA585', Aviation Accidents, 15 September 2017. <aviation-accidents.net/united-airlines-boeing-b737-200-n999ua-flight-ua585/>

Some of the surviving relatives of victims knew vaguely where the bodies were buried ... she said, 'Now I can die happily. Because now I know I'll see him, even in a bone, or an ash.': *The Silence of Others*, dir./prod. by Almudena Carracedo and Robert Bahar, El Deseo/Semilla Verde Productions/Lucernam Films, 2018. Broadcast on BBC's *Storyville* in December 2019.

Mendieta died a year after her father was found in the cemetery where he was shot: 'Ascensión Mendieta, 93, Dies: Symbol of Justice for Franco Victims', *New York Times*, 22 September 2019. <nytimes.com/2019/09/22/world/europe/ascension-mendieta-dies.html>

THE HORROR

a thirty-year-old computer programmer for Apple and Netscape named Thomas Dell, who ran the site anonymously under the pseudonym Soylent: Taylor Wofford, 'Rotten.com Is Offline', *The Outline*, 29 November 2017. <theoutline.com/post/2549/rotten-com-is-offline>

Though the photo was a fake, the sheer fact that he dared to publish it blew up in the global press: Janelle Brown, 'The Internet's Public

Enema No. 1', *Salon*, 5 March 2001. <salon.com/2001/03/05/rotten_2/>

'The gruesome invites us to be either spectators or cowards, unable to look': Susan Sontag, *Regarding the Pain of Others*, Penguin, London, 2003, p. 38.

The scene that changed everything for him was when Harvey Keitel turns up as Winston Wolfe: *Pulp Fiction*, written by Quentin Tarantino and Roger Avary, directed by Quentin Tarantino, Miramax Films, 1994. Reprinted by permission of Quentin Tarantino.

The detective in charge at the time described it to the *East Bay Times* as 'a takeover robbery, a real violent one': John Geluardi and Karl Fischer, 'Red Onion Owner Slain in Botched Takeover Robbery', *East Bay Times*, 28 April 2007. <eastbaytimes.com/2007/04/28/red-onion-owner-slain-in-botched-takeover-robbery/>

Andy Warhol was brought up a Catholic and was obsessed with images of death: Bradford R. Collins, 'Warhol's Modern Dance of Death', *American Art*, vol. 30, no. 2, University of Chicago Press, 2016, pp. 33–54. <journals.uchicago.edu/doi/full/10.1086/688590>

'The more you look at the same exact thing ... the more the meaning goes away, and the better and emptier you feel': Andy Warhol and Pat Hackett, *POPism: The Warhol Sixties*, Harper & Row, New York, 1980, p. 50 (in Collins, *Warhol*, p. 33).

'Sometimes he would say that he was scared of dying if he went to sleep ... So he'd lie in bed and listen to his heart beat': Henry Geldzahler, quoted in Jean Stein and George Plimpton, *Edie: An American Biography*, Alfred A. Knopf, New York, 1982, p. 201 (in Collins, *Warhol*, p. 37). Quoted with permission from the Plimpton Estate.

'Ever since cameras were invented in 1839, photography has kept company with death': Sontag, *Regarding the Pain of Others*, p. 21.

'Murder,' he said, 'is my business': Brian Wallis, *Weegee: Murder Is My Business*, International Center of Photography and DelMonico Books, New York, 2013, p. 9.

'I kept telling myself that I would believe the indescribably horrible sight in the courtyard': Margaret Bourke-White, *Dear Fatherland, Rest Quietly: A Report on the Collapse of Hitler's Thousand Years*, Arcole Publishing, Auckland, 2018.

Her photographs, published in LIFE magazine: Ben Cosgrove, 'Behind the Picture: The Liberation of Buchenwald, April 1945', *TIME*, 10 October 2013. <time.com/3638432/>

NOTES TO PAGES 97–107

Days later, the paper ran a notice saying the vulture was shooed away: 'Editor's Note', New York Times, 30 March 1993. <nytimes.com/1993/03/30/nyregion/editors-note-513893.html>

'I am haunted by the vivid memories of killings & corpses & anger & pain': Scott Macleod, 'The Life and Death of Kevin Carter', TIME, 24 June 2001. <content.time.com/time/magazine/article/0,9171,165071,00.html>

'compassion is an unstable emotion. It needs to be translated into action, or it withers ... One starts to get bored,' she says, 'cynical, apathetic': Sontag, Regarding the Pain of Others, pp. 90–1.

DINING WITH THE EXECUTIONER

this is the same state that, in 1992, saw then-governor Bill Clinton rush home from his presidential campaign trail to witness the execution of Ricky Ray Rector: Marc Mauer, 'Bill Clinton, "Black Lives" and the Myths of the 1994 Crime Bill', Marshall Project, 11 April 2016. <themarshallproject.org/2016/04/11/bill-clinton-black-lives-and-the-myths-of-the-1994-crime-bill>

In a letter dated 28 March 2017, signed by twenty-three former death row staff from across the nation: Letter to Governor Hutchinson, Constitution Project, 28 March 2017. <archive.constitutionproject.org/wp-content/uploads/2017/03/Letter-to-Governor-Hutchinson-from-Former-Corrections-Officials.pdf>

The licence plates on the vehicles in front of us say 'Virginia is for Lovers', all of them manufactured by inmates at a prison shop west of the city centre: Virginia Correctional Enterprises Tag Shop, Virginia Department of Corrections, YouTube, 12 April 2010. <youtu.be/SC-pzhP_kGc>

The United States was in the midst of a brief nationwide moratorium on capital punishment, bookended by two court cases: Robert Jay Lifton and Greg Mitchell, Who Owns Death? Capital Punishment, the American Conscience, and the End of Executions, HarperCollins, New York, 2000, pp. 40–1.

What is generally agreed to be the first American execution was carried out there in Jamestown: Ibid., p. 24.

In the state of New York, some were known to the public by name ... Others worked anonymously: Jennifer Gonnerman, 'The Last Executioner', Village Voice, 18 January 2005. <web.archive.org/web/20090612033107/http://www.villagevoice.com/2005-01-18/news/the-last-executioner/1>

The man who operated Florida's electric chair would already be wearing a hood: Lifton and Mitchell, *Who Owns Death?*, p. 88.

Florida was less covert than most and put out an ad for the job in the paper; they received twenty applications: Ibid.

Virginia's original electric chair, constructed by inmates in 1908 from an old oak tree: Deborah W. Denno, 'Is Electrocution an Unconstitutional Method of Execution? The Engineering of Death over the Century', *William & Mary Law Review*, vol. 35, no. 2, 1994, p. 648. <scholarship.law.wm.edu/wmlr/vol35/iss2/4>

according to one account by an attorney who was present, as a witness, as a representative to the General Assembly of Virginia, it did not go well: Ibid., p. 664.

He was the first to be executed by electrical current, if we don't count the old horse they tested the voltage on: Mark Essig, *Edison and the Electric Chair: A Story of Light and Death*, Sutton, Stroud, 2003, p. 225.

when the burned skin on his back was removed, the pathologist described his spinal muscles as looking like 'overcooked beef': 'Far Worse than Hanging: Kemmler's Death Provides an Awful Spectacle', *New York Times*, 7 August 1890. <timesmachine.nytimes.com/timesmachine/1890/08/07/103256332.pdf>

Sweat, however, is an excellent conductor: Katherine R. Notley, 'Virginia Death Row Inmates Sue to Stop Use of Electric Chair', *Executive Intelligence Review*, vol. 20, no. 9, 1993, p. 66. <larouchepub.com/eiw/public/1993/eirv20n09-19930226/eirv20n09-19930226_065-virginia_death_row_inmates_sue_t.pdf>

'whose touch was so profane that he could not come into contact with other people or objects without profoundly altering them': Paul Friedland, *Seeing Justice Done: The Age of Spectacular Capital Punishment in France*, Oxford University Press, 2012, pp. 71–2. Reproduced with permission of Oxford Publishing Ltd, the Licensor, through PLSclear.

'one of the most effective means of impugning someone's moral character was to insinuate that they had been seen dining with the executioner': Ibid., pp. 80–1.

Sometimes there are two switches pressed simultaneously and the machine decides which button will be live: Lifton and Mitchell, *Who Owns Death?*, p. 87.

Lewis E. Lawes, a warden at Sing Sing from 1920 to 1941, directed the execution of more than 200 men and women: Ibid., p. 102.

'the machinery of death cannot run without human hands to turn the dials': David R. Dow and Mark Dow, *Machinery of Death: The Reality of America's Death Penalty Regime*, Routledge, New York, 2002, p. 8. Reproduced with permission of Taylor and Francis Group LLC (Books) US, the Licensor, through PLSclear.

'We tell ourselves stories in order to live': Joan Didion, *The White Album*, Farrar, Straus and Giroux, New York, 2009, p. 11. Reprinted by permission of HarperCollins Publishers Ltd, © 1979 Joan Didion (UK).

Even the death squad leaders in the 1965 Indonesian genocide told themselves they were cool Hollywood gangsters: *The Act of Killing*, dir. Joshua Oppenheimer, Christine Cynn, Anonymous, Dogwoof Pictures, 2012.

statistically unproven idea of a deterrent: 'Deterrence: Studies Show No Link between the Presence or Absence of the Death Penalty and Murder Rates', Death Penalty Information Center. Last viewed 1 October 2021. <deathpenaltyinfo.org/policy-issues/deterrence>

short opinion pieces about decades of sleepless nights from former superintendents: S. Frank Thompson, 'I Know What It's Like to Carry Out Executions', *The Atlantic*, 3 December 2019. <theatlantic.com/ideas/archive/2019/12/federal-executions-trauma/602785/>

'I hope that the day is not far distant when legal slaying, whether by electrocution, hanging, lethal gas, or any other method is outlawed throughout the United States': Robert G. Elliott, *Agent of Death*, E. P. Dutton, New York, 1940.

Many have argued (Norman Mailer and Phil Donahue among them) that if America is serious about killing members of its public, then it should do so with a public audience: Christopher Hitchens, 'Scenes from an Execution', *Vanity Fair*, January 1998. <archive.vanityfair.com/article/share/3472d8c9-8efa-4989-b3da-72c7922cf70a>

Norman Mailer: Christopher Hitchens, 'A Minority of One: An Interview with Norman Mailer', *New Left Review*, no. 222, March/April 1997, pp. 7–9, 13. <newleftreview.org/issues/i222/articles/christopher-hitchens-norman-mailer-a-minority-of-one-an-interview-with-norman-mailer>

Phil Donahue: 'Donahue Cannot Film Execution', United Press International (UPI), 14 June 1994. <upi.com/Archives/1994/06/14/Donahue-cannot-film-execution/2750771566400/>

Albert Camus wrote about the guillotine: Albert Camus, *Resistance, Rebellion, and Death*, Alfred A. Knopf, New York, 1966, p. 175.

Jerry got a new job driving trucks for a company that installs guardrails along interstate highways: Dale Brumfield, 'An Executioner's Song', *Richmond Magazine*, 4 April 2016. <richmondmagazine.com/news/features/an-executioners-song/>

Morgan Freeman put him in his documentary series about God: 'Deadly Sins', Season 3, Episode 4 of *The Story of God with Morgan Freeman*, exec. prod. Morgan Freeman, Lori McCreary and James Younger, 2019, National Geographic Channel.

Dow B. Hover, a deputy sheriff, was the last person to serve as executioner in the state of New York … In 1990, he gassed himself in that same garage. John Hulbert, who served as New York's executioner from 1913 to 1926 … shot himself with a .38-calibre revolver: Jennifer Gonnerman, 'The Last Executioner', *The Village Voice*, 18 January 2005.

Donald Hocutt, who mixed the chemicals for the gas chamber in Mississippi, was haunted by nightmares: Lifton and Mitchell, *Who Owns Death?*, pp. 89–90.

'You've got five guys. One live round.': Jerry is slightly mistaken on the numbers here. Execution by firing squad involves five riflemen with four live rounds and one blank. Jerry's point, however, remains.

NONE OF THIS IS FOREVER

Twelve hours later the entire body is rigid: Val McDermid, *Forensics: The Anatomy of a Crime Scene*, Wellcome Collection, London, 2015, pp. 80–2.

in the case of the eccentric eighteenth-century British quack dentist Martin van Butchell: Susan Isaac, 'Martin Van Butchell: The Eccentric Dentist Who Embalmed His Wife', Royal College of Surgeons Library Blog, 1 March 2019. <www.rcseng.ac.uk/library-and-publications/library/blog/martin-van-butchell/>

But as the war escalated and the death toll mounted, bodies of soldiers – both Confederate and Union – overwhelmed hospital burial grounds: Drew Gilpin Faust, *This Republic of Suffering: Death and the American Civil War*, Vintage Civil War Library, New York, 2008, pp. 61–101.

Richer families would send for the bodies via the quartermaster general: Robert G. Mayer, *Embalming: History, Theory & Practice*, Third Edition, McGraw Hill, New York, 2000, p. 464.

when a young colonel called Elmer Ellsworth – formerly employed as a law clerk in President Lincoln's hometown office – was shot and killed as he seized a Confederate flag: Faust, *Suffering*, p. 94.

French inventor, Jean-Nicolas Gannal, whose book – detailing his method of preserving bodies for anatomical study: Anne Carol, 'Embalming and Materiality of Death: France, Nineteenth Century', *Mortality*, vol. 24, no. 2, 2019, pp.183–92. <tandfonline.com/doi/full/10.1080/13576275.2019.1585784>

In his shopfront in Washington DC, he displayed the body of an unknown man: Faust, *Suffering*, p. 95.

the US Army received complaints from families saying they had been cheated by embalmers: Ibid., pp. 96–7.

One embalmer in Puerto Rico has since taken it to an extreme, posing bodies like statues at their own wakes: Nick Kirkpatrick, 'A Funeral Home's Specialty: Dioramas of the (Propped Up) Dead', *Washington Post*, 27 May 2014. <washingtonpost.com/news/morning-mix/wp/2014/05/27/a-funeral-homes-specialty-dioramas-of-the-propped-up-dead/>

'the ugly facts are relentlessly hidden; the art of embalmers is an art of complete denial': Geoffrey Gorer, 'The Pornography of Death', *Encounter*, October 1955, pp. 49–52.

'donning the mantle of the psychiatrist when it suits their purposes': Jessica Mitford, *The American Way of Death Revisited*, Virago, London, 2000, p. 64. Reproduced with the permission of the Jessica Mitford heirs.

I had described the physical process of embalming as 'violent' in a magazine article: Campbell, 'In the future …', *WIRED*.

between 50 per cent and 55 per cent of bodies in the UK are embalmed in a typical year: Email exchange with Karen Caney FBIE, National General Secretary, British Institute of Embalmers.

Those embalmed men returned from the Civil War continue to leach arsenic – a long-ago outlawed ingredient – into the soil around them: Mollie Bloudoff-Indelicato, 'Arsenic and Old Graves: Civil War-Era Cemeteries May Be Leaking Toxins', *Smithsonian Magazine*, 30 October 2015. <smithsonianmag.com/science-nature/arsenic-and-old-graves-civil-war-era-cemeteries-may-be-leaking-toxins-180957115/>

These days in the US, more than 3 million litres of embalming fluid, complete with carcinogenic formaldehyde, are buried every year: Green Burial Council, 'Disposition Statistics', via Mary Woodsen of Cornell University and Greensprings Natural Preserve in Newfield,

New York. Last viewed 1 October 2021. <greenburialcouncil.org/media_packet.html>

In 2015, flooding in cemeteries in Northern Ireland brought the chemicals to the surface: Malachi O'Doherty, 'Toxins Leaking from Embalmed Bodies in Graveyards Pose Threat to the Living', *Belfast Telegraph*, 10 May 2015. <belfasttelegraph.co.uk/news/northern-ireland/toxins-leaking-from-embalmed-bodies-in-graveyards-pose-threat-to-the-living-31211012.html>

In Tana Toraja, Indonesia, families periodically take the dead out of their tombs to wash and dress them: Caitlin Doughty, *From Here to Eternity*, W.W. Norton, New York, 2017, pp. 42–77.

LOVE AND TERROR

the infant mortality rate in the UK is, while falling, still higher than other comparable countries: 'How Does the UK's Infant Mortality Rate Compare Internationally?', Nuffield Trust, 29 July 2021. <nuffieldtrust.org.uk/resource/infant-and-neonatal-mortality>

an English soap star campaigned for foetuses born dead before a certain age to have birth certificates as well as death certificates: Seamus Duff and Ellie Henman, 'Law Changer: Kym Marsh Relives Heartache of Her Son's Tragic Death as She Continues Campaign to Change Law for Those Who Give Birth and Lose Their Baby', *The Sun*, 31 January 2017. <thesun.co.uk/tvandshowbiz/2745250/kym-marsh-relives-heartache-of-her-sons-tragic-death-as-she-continues-campaign-to-change-law-for-those-who-give-birth-and-lose-their-baby/>

'the corpse, seen without God and outside of science, is the utmost of abjection. It is death infecting life': Julia Kristeva, *Powers of Horror: An Essay on Abjection*, Columbia University Press, New York, 1980, p. 4. Reproduced with permission of Columbia University Press.

Maggie Rae, president of the Faculty of Public Health, was quoted in the *British Medical Journal*: Matthew Limb, 'Disparity in Maternal Deaths because of Ethnicity is "Unacceptable"', *The BMJ*, 18 January 2021. <bmj.com/content/372/bmj.n152>

TOUGH MOTHER

they were self-appointed carers during pregnancy and birth: 'Tracing Midwives in Your Family', Royal College of Obstetricians

& Gynaecologists/Royal College of Midwives, 2014. <rcog.org.uk/
globalassets/documents/guidelines/library-services/heritage/rcm-
genealogy.pdf>

lay out the dead: 'How Do You Lay Someone Out When They Die?', Funeral
Guide, 22 February 2018. <funeralguide.co.uk/blog/laying-out-a-
body>

**only 12 per cent of neonatal units have mandatory bereavement
training**: 'Audit of Bereavement Care Provision in UK Neonatal
Units 2018', Sands, 2018. <sands.org.uk/audit-bereavement-care-
provision-uk-neonatal-units-2018>

**it is estimated that one in every four pregnancies ends in loss during
pregnancy or birth. One in every 250 pregnancies ends in stillbirth; eight babies are stillborn across the UK every day**: 'Pregnancy
Loss Statistics', Tommy's. Last viewed 1 October 2021. <tommys.org/
our-organisation/our-research/pregnancy-loss-statistics>

**fewer than half of the women who experience a miscarriage ever find
out why it happened**: 'Tell Me Why', Tommy's. Last viewed 1 October
2021. <tommys.org/our-research/tell-me-why>

**Ariel Levy talks about the miscarriage she had at five months on the
bathroom floor in a hotel in Mongolia**: Ariel Levy, 'Thanksgiving
in Mongolia', New Yorker, 10 November 2013. <newyorker.com/maga-
zine/2013/11/18/thanksgiving-in-mongolia> Text from this article
was reproduced in her book: Ariel Levy, The Rules Do Not Apply, Random
House, New York, 2017/Fleet, London, 2017, pp. 145–6, 235–6.
Reproduced with permission of Penguin Random House LLC (US).

**of the 377 women spoken to whose babies were stillborn or died
soon after birth**: Katherine J. Gold, Irving Leon, Martha E. Boggs and
Ananda Sen, 'Depression and Posttraumatic Stress Symptoms after
Perinatal Loss in a Population-Based Sample', Journal of Women's Health,
vol. 25, no. 3, 2016, pp. 263–8. <ncbi.nlm.nih.gov/pmc/articles/
PMC4955602/pdf/jwh.2015.5284.pdf>

THE DEVIL'S COACHMAN

**the cremation rate in the UK has risen from around 35 per cent to
78 per cent of all funerals (America is lagging behind at 55 per
cent)**: 'International Statistics 2019', Cremation Society. Last viewed 1
October 2021. <cremation.org.uk/International-cremation-statistics-
2019>

'blind, emotionless alien': Christopher Hitchens, *Mortality*, Atlantic Books, London, 2012, p. 11. Reproduced with permission from Atlantic Books Ltd (UK) and Hachette Book Group (USA).

THE HOPEFUL DEAD

The mayor tried to get those that stayed to move further in: Jonathan Oosting, 'Detroit Mayor Dave Bing: Relocation "Absolutely" Part of Plan to Downsize City', Michigan Live, 25 February 2010. <mlive. com/news/detroit/2010/02/detroit_mayor_dave_bing_reloca. html>

even Benjamin Franklin suggested something similar in 1773: Ed Regis, *Great Mambo Chicken and the Transhumanist Condition: Science Slightly Over the Edge*, Perseus Books, New York, 1990, p. 84.

Fiction was, after all, where he had come across the idea originally: Ibid., p. 85.

'Only those embrace death who are half dead already': Robert Ettinger, *The Prospect of Immortality*, Sidgwick & Jackson, London, 1965, p. 146.

Alcor in Arizona, at $200,000: Alcor, Membership/Funding. Last viewed 1 October 2021. <alcor.org/membership/>

how the bodies of his frozen clients were stored in a garage behind a mortuary: Sam Shaw, 'Mistakes Were Made: You're as Cold as Ice', *This American Life*, episode 354, 18 April 2008. <thisamericanlife.org/354/ mistakes-were-made>

recently reanimated organisms: David Wallace-Wells, *The Uninhabitable Earth*, Allen Lane, London, 2019, p. 99.

researchers had, in 2019, taken the brains out of the heads of thirty-two dead pigs: Gina Kolata, '"Partly Alive": Scientists Revive Cells in Brains from Dead Pigs', *New York Times*, 17 April 2019. <nytimes. com/2019/04/17/science/brain-dead-pigs.html>

In the frogs, as the temperature drops, special proteins in their blood suck the water out of the cells: John Roach, 'Antifreeze-Like Blood Lets Frogs Freeze and Thaw with Winter's Whims', *National Geographic*, 20 February 2007. <nationalgeographic.com/animals/2007/02/ frog-antifreeze-blood-winter-adaptation/>

AFTERWORD

'Burnout is more than an occupational hazard in the homicide unit, it is a psychological certainty': David Simon, *Homicide: A Year on the*

Killing Streets, Houghton Mifflin Company, Boston, 1991, p. 177. © David Simon, 1991, 2006. Extracts from *Homicide: A Year on the Killing Streets* reproduced with permission of Canongate Books Ltd and Henry Holt & Co.

'However, stress hormones are meant to give us the strength and endurance to respond to extraordinary conditions': Bessel van der Kolk, *The Body Keeps the Score*, Penguin, London, 2014, p. 217. Reproduced with permission of Penguin Random House LLC (US). Reprinted by permission of Penguin Books Ltd. (UK), © 2014 Bessel van der Kolk.

'the two incommensurate human emotions strike and collide': Richard Powers, introduction to DeLillo, *White Noise*, pp. xi–xii. Reproduced with permission of Penguin Random House LLC (US).

a single image of a dead Chinese man: Agence France-Presse, 'A Man Lies Dead in the Street: The Image that Captures the Wuhan Coronavirus Crisis', *Guardian*, 31 January 2020. <theguardian.com/world/2020/jan/31/a-man-lies-dead-in-the-street-the-image-that-captures-the-wuhan-coronavirus-crisis>

'The more remote or exotic the place, the more likely we are to have full frontal views of the dead and dying': Sontag, *Regarding the Pain of Others*, p. 63.

650 bodies on the Brooklyn waterfront: Paul Berger, 'NYC Dead Stay in Freezer Trucks Set Up during Spring Covid-19 Surge', *Wall Street Journal*, 22 November 2020. <wsj.com/articles/nyc-dead-stay-in-freezer-trucks-set-up-during-spring-covid-19-surge-11606050000>

Los Angeles county temporarily suspended air-quality regulations: Julia Carrie Wong, 'Los Angeles Lifts Air-Quality Limits for Cremations as Covid Doubles Death Rate', *Guardian*, 18 January 2021. <theguardian.com/us-news/2021/jan/18/los-angeles-covid-coronavirus-deaths-cremation-pandemic>

In Brazil, when the daily death toll spilled over 4,000, nurses on Covid isolation wards filled nitrile gloves with warm water: 'Nursing Technician from São Carlos "Supports" an Intubated Patient's Hand with Gloves Filled with Warm Water', Globo.com, 23 March 2021. <g1.globo.com/sp/sao-carlos-regiao/noticia/2021/03/23/tecnica-em-enfermagem-de-sao-carlos-ampara-mao-de-paciente-intubada-com-luvas-cheias-de-agua-morna.ghtml>

'I wish we could have our old life back. We had the greatest economy that we've ever had, and we didn't have death': *Remarks by President*

Trump, Vice President Pence, and Members of the Coronavirus Task Force in Press Briefing, issued on 30 March 2020, press briefing held 29 March 2020, 5.43 p.m. EDT. <trumpwhitehouse.archives.gov/briefings-statements/remarks-president-trump-vice-president-pence-members-coronavirus-task-force-press-briefing-14/

Further Reading

DEATH/DYING

Alvarez, Al, *The Savage God: A Study of Suicide*, Bloomsbury, London, 2002.

Ariès, Philippe, *The Hour of Our Death: The Classic History of Western Attitudes toward Death over the Last One Thousand Years*, Alfred A. Knopf, New York, 1981.

Becker, Ernest, *The Denial of Death*, The Free Press, New York, 1973.

Callender, Ru, Lara Dinius-Inman, Rosie Inman-Cook, Michael Jarvis, Dr John Mallatratt, Susan Morris, Judith Pidgeon and Brett Walwyn, *The Natural Death Handbook*, The Natural Death Centre, Winchester, and Strange Attractor Press, London, 2012.

Critchley, Simon, *Notes on Suicide*, Fitzcarraldo Editions, London, 2015.

Doughty, Caitlin, *Smoke Gets In Your Eyes, and Other Lessons from the Crematory*, W.W. Norton, New York, 2014.

——, *From Here to Eternity*, W.W. Norton, New York, 2017.

Gawande, Atul, *Being Mortal: Illness, Medicine, and What Matters in the End*, Profile Books, London, 2014.

Hitchens, Christopher, *Mortality*, Atlantic Books, London, 2012.

Jarman, Derek, *Modern Nature: The Journals of Derek Jarman 1989–1990*, Vintage, London, 1991.

Kalanithi, Paul, *When Breath Becomes Air*, The Bodley Head, London, 2016.

Kristeva, Julia, *Powers of Horror: An Essay on Abjection*, Columbia University Press, New York, 1980.

Kübler-Ross, Elisabeth, *On Death and Dying: What the Dying Have to Teach Doctors, Nurses, Clergy and Their Own Families*, Scribner, New York, 1969.

Laqueur, Thomas W., *The Work of the Dead: A Cultural History of Mortal Remains*, Princeton University Press, Princeton, NJ, 2015.

Lesy, Michael, *The Forbidden Zone*, André Deutsch, London, 1988.

Lofland, Lyn H., *The Craft of Dying: The Modern Face of Death*, Sage, Los Angeles, 1978.

Mitford, Jessica, *The American Way of Death Revisited*, Virago, London, 2000.

Nuland, Sherwin B., *How We Die*, Vintage, London, 1993.

O'Mahony, Seamus, *The Way We Die Now*, Head of Zeus, London, 2016.

Terkel, Studs, *Will the Circle Be Unbroken? Reflections on Death, Rebirth, and Hunger for a Faith*, New York Press, New York, 2001.

Troyer, John, *Technologies of the Human Corpse*, MIT Press, Cambridge, MA, 2020.

Wojnarowicz, David, *Close to the Knives: A Memoir of Disintegration*, Canongate, Edinburgh, 2017.

Yalom, Irvin D., *Existential Psychotherapy*, Basic Books, New York, 1980.

AFTERMATH

Black, Sue, *All that Remains: A Life in Death*, Doubleday, London, 2018.

Didion, Joan, *The Year of Magical Thinking*, Fourth Estate, London, 2012.

Ernaux, Annie, *Happening*, Fitzcarraldo Editions, London, 2019.

Faust, Drew Gilpin, *This Republic of Suffering: Death and the American Civil War*, Vintage Civil War Library, New York, 2008.

Lloyd Parry, Richard, *Ghosts of the Tsunami*, Vintage, London, 2017.

ANATOMISTS/DISSECTION

Blakely, Robert L., and Judith M. Harrington, *Bones in the Basement: Postmortem Racism in Nineteeth-Century Medical Training*, Smithsonian Institution Press, Washington, 1997.

Fitzharris, Lindsey, *The Butchering Art*, Farrar, Straus, and Giroux, New York, 2017.

Moore, Wendy, *The Knife Man: Blood, Body-Snatching and the Birth of Modern Surgery*, Bantam, London, 2005.

Park, Katharine, *Secrets of Women: Gender, Generation, and the Origins of Human Dissection*, Zone Books, New York, 2010.

Richardson, Ruth, *Death, Dissection and the Destitute*, Penguin, London, 1988.

Rifkin, Benjamin A., Michael J. Ackerman, and Judith Folkenberg, *Human Anatomy: Depicting the Body from the Renaissance to Today*, Thames & Hudson, London, 2006.

Roach, Mary, *Stiff: The Curious Lives of Human Cadavers*, Penguin, New York, 2003.

Shelley, Mary, *Frankenstein*, Penguin, London, 1992. (First published 1818.)

Worden, Gretchen, *Mütter Museum of the College of Physicians of Philadelphia*, Blast Books, New York, 2002.

CRIME

Botz, Corinne May, *The Nutshell Studies of Unexplained Death*, The Monacelli Press, New York, 2004.

McDermid, Val, *Forensics: The Anatomy of Crime*, Profile Books, London, 2015.

Nelson, Maggie, *The Red Parts: Autobiography of a Trial*, Vintage, London, 2017.

Simon, David, *Homicide: A Year on the Killing Streets*, Houghton Mifflin Company, Boston, 1991.

IMAGES OF DEATH

Benkard, Ernst, *Undying Faces*, Hogarth Press, London, 1929.

Ebenstein, Joanna, *Death: A Graveside Companion*, Thames & Hudson, London, 2017.

Friedrich, Ernst, *War against War!*, Spokesman, Nottingham, 2014 (facsimile edition of 1924 publication).

Heyert, Elizabeth, *The Travelers*, Scalo, Zürich, 2006.

Koudounaris, Paul, *Memento Mori: The Dead Among Us*, Thames & Hudson, London, 2015.

Marinovich, Greg, and João Silva, *The Bang-Bang Club: Snapshots from a Hidden War*, Arrow, London, 2001.

Sontag, Susan, *Regarding the Pain of Others*, Penguin, London, 2003.

Thanatos Archive, *Beyond the Dark Veil: Post-Mortem & Mourning Photography*, Grand Central Press & Last Gasp, California, 2015.

Wallis, Brian, *Weegee: Murder Is My Business*, International Center of Photography and DelMonico Books, New York, 2013.

CAPITAL PUNISHMENT

Cabana, Donald A., *Death at Midnight: The Confession of an Executioner*, Northeastern University Press, Boston, 1996.

Camus, Albert, *Resistance, Rebellion, and Death*, Alfred A. Knopf, New York, 1966.

Dow, David R., and Mark Dow, *Machinery of Death: The Reality of America's Death Penalty Regime*, Routledge, New York, 2002.

Edds, Margaret, *An Expendable Man: The Near-Execution of Earl Washington, Jr.*, New York University Press, New York, 2003.

Koestler, Arthur, *Dialogue With Death: The Journal of a Prisoner of the Fascists in the Spanish Civil War*, The University of Chicago Press, Chicago, 2011.

Lifton, Robert Jay, and Greg Mitchell, *Who Owns Death? Capital Punishment, the American Conscience, and the End of Executions*, HarperCollins, New York, 2000.

Solotaroff, Ivan, *The Last Face You'll Ever See: The Private Life of the American Death Penalty*, HarperCollins, New York, 2001.

CEMETERIES

Arnold, Catharine, *Necropolis: London and Its Dead*, Simon & Schuster, London, 2006.

Beesley, Ian, and David James, *Undercliffe: Bradford's Historic Victorian Cemetery*, Ryburn Publishing, Halifax, 1991.

Harrison, Robert Pogue, *The Dominion of the Dead*, University of Chicago Press, Chicago, 2003.

Swannell, John, *Highgate Cemetery*, Hurtwood Press, Oxted, 2010.

CRYONICS

Ettinger, Robert C. W., *The Prospect of Immortality*, Sidgwick & Jackson, London, 1965.

Nelson, Robert F. and Sandra Stanley, *We Froze the First Man: The Startling True Story of the First Great Step toward Human Immortality*, Dell, New York, 1968.

O'Connell, Mark, *To Be a Machine*, Granta, London, 2017.

FOR KIDS

Erlbruch, Wolf, *Death, Duck and the Tulip*, Gecko Press, Minneapolis, 2008.

Index

embalming, 16, 24–5, 37, 39–40, 54,
123–6, 129–47
and cryonics, 213, 216, 220
embalming fluids, 24–5, 93, 137–8,
140–3, 215
epilepsy, 155
ethyl mercaptan, 20
Ettinger, Robert, 206–9, 212, 218
euphemisms, 131
European Broadcasting Union, 236
euthanasia, 215
Everglades National Park, 42
executions, 31, 56, 58, 94, 101–
3, 106–21
eye caps, 135–6
eyebrows, 145

faces, 45–6, 55, 84, 200
Falklands War, 60
Farley, Chris, 87
feet, 46
fentanyl, 18
Figueroa, Alfredo, 91
fingerprints, 53, 71–2, 75, 77–8, 85
firing squads, 120–1
Fisher, Dean, 28
Fixodent, 159, 162
fly prints, 92, 99
formaldehyde, 37, 137–8
Francel, Joseph, 120
Francis, Pope, 73
Franco, General Francisco, 80
Frankenstein, 32, 211
Franklin, Aretha, 132
Franklin, Benjamin, 207
Fraser, 'Mad' Frankie, 59
Freeman, Morgan, 119
Friedland, Paul, 110–11
Futurama, 41, 208

Gabor, Zsa Zsa, 206
gag reflex, 92
Gannal, Jean-Nicolas, 124
gardening, 236–237

Geldzahler, Henry, 94–5
genetic counselling, 167
Germanwings, 64, 70
ghosts, 199
Givens, Jerry, 102–21, 223, 230
Gladstone, William, 84, 233
Good, Daniel, 58
Gore, Dr Philip, 130–4, 140, 144–6
Gorer, Geoffrey, 125
gravediggers, 188–91
Great Train Robbery, 49, 58
Greeks, ancient, 51
Grenfell Tower, 67–8, 83
Gross, Terry, 235
guillotine, 111, 118

hands, 41, 77
Harrington rods, 38
Harvey, William, 31
heads, removal of, 43
heart bypass valves, 38
Heartlands Hospital, 172
hearts, weighing, 149, 157
Henry VIII, King, 30
hepatitis, 25
Hepworth, Barbara, 12
Highgate Cemetery, 50, 61–2, 126
hip replacement, 38–9
Hitchens, Christopher, 203
HMS Hermes, 60
hoarding, 92
Hocutt, Donald, 120
Holmes, Thomas, 124
homeless people, 76
homosexuality, 10
Horsley, Sebastian, 52
hospice movement, 127
Hover, Dow B., 120
Hugo, Victor, 50
Hulbert, John, 120
humectants, 25
Hunter, John, 31, 41
Hunter, William, 31, 35
Hunterian Museum, 31–2, 41

Acknowledgements

Thank you to all the dead I met whose names I know and those I don't.

Thank you also to the living, for their time and their work: Poppy Mardall, Aaron and Roseanna in the mortuary, Terry Regnier, Nick Reynolds, Mark "Mo" Oliver, Neal Smither, Jerry Givens, Ron and Jean Troyer, Dr Philip Gore, Kevin Sinclair, Lara-Rose Iredale, Clare Beesley, Mike and Bob at Arnos Vale, Tony and Dave at Canford Crematorium, Dennis and Hillary at the Cryonics Institute, and Anthony Mattick.

Thank you to Clint Edwards, my first and closest reader, my lighthouse when I was lost in a sea of transcripts and drafts, my trusty driver of shitty rental cars, and the poor bastard who lived through not only several painful deadlines with me but also a global pandemic: Wayne and Waynetta forever. Eddie Campbell and Audrey Niffenegger, my favourite couple of weirdos, without whom there might have been no book at all. Kristofor Minta, for introducing me to Ernest Becker all those years ago and dealing with what came next. Caitlin Doughty, for her wisdom and a place to crash (sorry I attempted to grind coffee beans in your milkshake blender). Dr John Troyer, overlord of death, for opening doors and letting me borrow his brains and his family. Sally Orson-Jones, for arguing with me until I figured out what I was trying to say. Oli Franklin-Wallis, for the pep talks on the ledge. Cat Mihos, my lab rat (apologies in addition to thank yous).

Thank you to the kind, patient and smart people at Raven Books, most of all Alison Hennessey and Katie Ellis-Brown, as well as Hannah Phillips at St. Martin's Press. Thank you to my agents Laura Macdougall, Olivia Davies, Sulamita Garbuz, and Jon Elek. Thank you also to The Society of Authors and the Authors' Foundation for partially funding this thing.

There are numerous people who answered my seemingly random questions – whether about birds, letter carving, or consciousness – or somehow helped along the way. Thank you to Professor Dame Sue Black, Vivienne McGuire at the Centre for Anatomy and Human Identification at the University of Dundee, Paul Kefford, Dean Fisher at UCLA, Roger Avary, Anil Seth, BJ Miller, Bryan Magee, Bruce Levine, Eric Marland, Sharon Stiteler, Nick Booth, Rabbi Laura Janner-Klausner, Lucy Coleman Talbot, João Medeiros, Dr Ollie Minton and Vanessa Spencer at Arnos Vale.

This book was written at the back of a bus in rural Minnesota, next to a tumble dryer in a New York hotel that is now in the process of being demolished, on a rooftop in New Orleans and typed in a car outside an Arby's somewhere in Michigan, but mostly it was written in North London. Thank you to my pals who variously gave me places to sleep, lifts, books, dinner, all of the above or simply an invitation to air my grievances: Eleanor Morgan, Olly Richards, Leo Barker, Nathaniel Metcalfe, Ossie Hirst, Andy Riley and Polly Faber, Cate Sevilla, Neil Gaiman, Amanda Palmer, Bill Stiteler, Stephen Rodrick, Toby Finlay, Darren Richman, Tom Spurgeon who rescued us one snowy night in Ohio (rest in peace, old friend), Erin and Mackenzie Dalrymple, Michael and Courtney Gaiman, and my own personal George Costanza, John Saward. Thank you to Peter and Jackie Knight for looking after Ned the cat, and thank you to Ned himself: my shadow, my paperweight, my self-appointed alarm clock.

Writing this book made my hair streak grey, so thank you to Susan Sontag and Lily Munster for making it look deliberate.

A Note on the Author

Hayley Campbell is an author, broadcaster and journalist. Her work has appeared in *WIRED*, *The Guardian*, *New Statesman*, *Empire*, and more. She lives in London with her cat, Ned.